Leila Mary Costin

# LIVING MEDICINE

A guide to those plants that have been scientifically
proved to have healing properties, showing how to
recognize them, when best to pick them, and how
to prepare them for medicinal use.

# LIVING MEDICINE
## The Healing Properties of Plants

*by*

MANNFRIED PAHLOW
Introduction by Dr Karl Heinz Caspers

Translated from the German by
Linda Sonntag

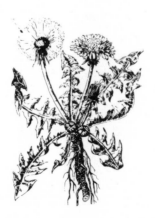

THORSONS PUBLISHERS LIMITED
Wellingborough, Northamptonshire

First published in Germany as *Heilpflanzen heute*
© 1976 Gräfe und Unzer GmbH, München
First published in England 1980


© THORSONS PUBLISHERS LIMITED 1980

ISBN 0 7225 0592 2 (paperback)
ISBN 0 7225 0605 8 (hardback)


Typeset by Harper Phototypesetters, Northampton.
Printed in Great Britain by Lowe and Brydone Printers Ltd.,
Thetford, Norfolk, and bound by
Weatherby Woolnough, Wellingborough, Northamptonshire.

# CONTENTS

# INTRODUCTION

Today no-one wants to follow blindly the recipes of quack doctors or listen uncritically to the tales of old wives when it comes to the use of plants in medicine. People are not so credulous as to believe that the woods and fields abound with common plants that will miraculously cure their every ailment, and their scepticism will not be brushed aside by the old wive's tale that what doesn't cure you won't kill you either.

For everybody who wants to know the real facts about the medicinal properties of plants, we have written this modern guide to plant remedies: a book which combines the latest scientific discoveries with the knowledge gained from years of experience in pharmacy. Old traditional recipes for teas and infusions, the potency of which has been proved by scientific investigation, are included alongside more up-to-date remedies; but plants which had wondrous healing powers ascribed to them which they do not possess are not.

The aim of the book is to restore people's trust in the healing power of plants. Plants are a valuable source of natural medicine which can have remarkable curative effects, provided that they are put to the correct use. This book will show you how.

The Catalogue of Healing Plants contains only those plants which can safely be used by the layman without danger to his health. The reader will learn the reasons why certain plants cure certain ailments, and exactly how to prepare and use them for the best effects.

While the pharmaceutical industry harvests huge plantations of healing plants for use in the production of drugs each year, we should not forget that the woods and fields offer a rich supply of natural and *free* remedies to the informed collector. Here plants, roots, blossoms and berries can be freshly gathered according to the Collector's Calendar (page 37) which gives advice on location, harvesting time and methods of culling and storage.

The final chapter deals with exotic plants and plants with newly discovered powers, such as garlic, ginseng and devil's claw, which are much talked about today for their 'magical' qualities. It also covers plants so potent that they should be taken only on the advice of a qualified practitioner. These can be as dangerous as any mass-produced drug used wrongly, and should therefore be avoided in self-treatment.

# CHAPTER ONE

# THE ROLE OF PLANTS IN MODERN MEDICINE

Plants are an intrinsic part of natural medicine, and not even the most orthodox doctor can get by without them; indeed they represent the link between the natural and the orthodox, the traditional and the ultra-new. Take for example the common foxglove. From this we get digitalis, a healing agent whose derivatives are used in the most advanced treatment of heart disease.

But, though plants span both worlds of medicine, their natural home is in natural therapy, for both historical and practical reasons.

**What is natural therapy?**
To many people natural therapy is synonymous with herbal remedies bought from health shops, but there is more to it than this. The essence of natural therapy is to activate the body's own self-healing powers. In other words, natural therapy is the administration of a natural remedy, which allows the body to cure itself. The body's natural healing powers are part of the life force which runs through every living being, and these are at the centre of natural medicine.

However, to use the terms 'natural healing powers' and 'life force' is to tread on dangerous ground, for both expressions, once so respectable, have been bandied about and misused over the years to the point where serious doctors and scientists will no longer give them credit. On the other hand, no-one would disagree that there are forms of energy which create and maintain life, and which restore the diseased to health. As long as the terms 'natural healing powers' and 'life force' refer to this and nothing else, their validity will not be disputed.

From the beginning of time it has been the doctor's job to activate these natural forces, without which all his medicine would be in vain. Medicine cannot *change* the workings of the body, it can only *help* them. One of the oldest medical teachings says *'medicus cura, natura sanat':* in other words, the doctor treats, but nature heals.

This principle seems so simple that the layman will have no problem in accepting it. Yet the specialist, who has been trained for years in science or medicine, will often forget that it is true, and attribute absolute powers of healing to technology. Many doctors believe that their patients get well because of drugs and surgery alone, and ignore the fact that the body has its own healing powers. To them therapy is merely the administration of treatment: medicine is poured into the body as if it were an empty vessel devoid of life.

This is chemistry, not healing! Of course this method has its uses, especially in cases of emergency when the patient's life depends on immediate and drastic treatment, but whether its beneficial effects are long-lasting is another question. Does it really help a patient worn down by a long and serious illness? And what does it do for someone who is feeling merely 'under the weather'?

It goes without saying that the whole of modern medicine doesn't ascribe to this mechanistic viewpoint, but there certainly are doctors who regard nature as an enemy rather than as a friend.

The life force gave us life in the first place and it is this which delivers us from disease until the day when it is finally extinguished in us. As such it is the doctor's greatest ally in his most important task: to help the human body help itself.

### Natural healing

Natural healing is becoming increasingly popular today and many people are turning to alternative treatments like acupuncture, homoeopathy and radionics, which they find can help them where orthodox medicine has failed.

An important principle in the application of all these aids is that natural medicine regards man as an entity, not just an assemblage of parts. Thus treatment is aimed at the whole man and not, as in orthodox medicine, merely at the part that has gone wrong. A patient treated with natural healing aids will not necessarily recover very quickly, but once he is back on his feet he will feel stronger than if he had been taking ordinary medicine. In all probability he will find that it takes him less time to convalesce, too.

The 'quick recovery from 'flu treated with antibiotics, and the ensuing period, often lasting for months, when the patient feels neither well nor ill, is known to most of us. And this is the reason for another of the principles of natural medicine: all things should be allowed to take their natural course.

Natural medicine never takes a hammer to crack a nut: it employs methods and means of healing that are just as strong as is necessary for recovery. The body needs support and the stimulus to heal itself: bombarding it with medicine gives it neither of these.

### Plants and homoeopathy

Plants are used extensively in homoeopathy, an alternative medicine very different from plant medicine, the modern principles which were founded about 150 years ago by Dr Samuel Hahnemann. In homoeopathy the plant material used is determined after a very thorough investigation of the patient and his way of life. It is made into a solution and diluted many times over, so that only a minute amount of the original substance remains. Paradoxically, this dilution represents an increase of the healing properties of the plant. The principle behind homoeopathy is to stimulate the body into reacting defensively for its own good. The minute dosage of the healing agent triggers off a response in the body opposite to that given by a large dosage of the same agent. Here is an example. The homoeopathic remedy for insomnia is a preparation made from a high dilution of caffeine, which is taken from the coffee plant. Coffee it is well known, is normally given (but not in dilution) for the opposite purpose, namely to keep someone awake. So the same agent can act as a stimulant when taken in large doses, and as a soporific when taken diluted.

Homoeopathy thus treats like with like (Greek: *homoeo*-like), using plant remedies which, when given to a healthy person, cause symptoms of the very disease they are used to cure. Plant medicine uses substances which produce exactly the opposite effect, admittedly without diluting them. To treat insomnia it would not use caffeine, a stimulant, but a soporific such as balm or hops. Thus plant medicine belongs to allopathy (Greek: *allos*-other). The only similarity between homoeopathy and herbal medicine is that both make use of plants and both belong under the umbrella of natural medicine.

## Plants and orthodox medicine

Plants are used as therapeutic agents in every branch of orthodox medicine. Basically, they are employed in three ways:

1. As a drug or preparation which contains *all* the substances of a certain part (fruit, leaves, root etc.) of a given plant.
2. In a refined or purified form or as a standardized extract.
3. As a derivative, which will contain certain elements present in the plant combined chemically with other synthetic substances.

Each of these forms can also be found combined with other, mostly synthetic substances, and all are employed according to the principles of orthodox medicine, namely allopathically and in a manner governed by the symptoms of the disease.

## Healing and health

Before turning to the healing plants themselves, it is worth considering the meaning of the words 'healing' and 'health', both to get closer to the mind of the doctor and to understand what to expect, and what not to expect, from herbal remedies.

The word 'heal' comes from the Gothic *hailjan,* to make whole, and hence 'health' means wholeness. But those whose business it is to 'make whole' have never been known to agree on an exact definition of what the condition of wholeness is. Some talk scientifically of health as normality, and set themselves standards to measure it by, while others withdraw lamely behind a less positive statement: health is the absence of illness. Still others go further and bring both body and soul into their definition, and the World Health Organization has reached a formula which is as desirable as it is idealistic: 'Health is the condition of perfect bodily, spiritual and social wellbeing and not solely the absence of illness and injury'.

This book is not the place to discuss the political and economical implications of such a Utopian statement, but it must be seen that the variety of definitions which exist does nothing to ease the confusion of the doctor whose job it is to produce this mysterious condition, 'health'. Each doctor has to make up his own mind as to the meaning of the word.

If he decides that his job is solely to restore the (subjective) wellbeing of his patient, his treatment will be symptomatic and he will lower a patient's temperature or suppress a cough. He may on the other hand decide to treat the causes, rather than the symptoms, of an illness; the general rather than the particular. In this case he could decide to let a fever run its course, or even to induce one, or to restore the energy balance of the body by acupuncture or other similar means. Alternatively, he could treat bodily disorders and injuries (such as stomach ulcers) by harmonizing the disturbed relationship between body and soul. This would involve the patient in a pro-

gramme of spiritual relaxation through a discipline such as meditation or yoga.

The type of treatment that a doctor prescribes will depend very much on his own definition of the word 'health'. This definition can't be changed to suit the patient or the disease, but must be made once and for all and applied to every case and every situation. Admittedly, a doctor can change his ideas about health several times in the course of his career, but each time he does, he makes his allegiance to a different method of treatment and a different school of thought.

Doctors haven't always had this decision to make. There was only one kind of medicine until a little over a hundred years ago, when the eminent pathologist Virchow discovered cellular differentiation and split the medical world into two factions: the general doctor and the specialist.

Medical students were taught more and more to specialize and concentrate on particular areas (like ear, nose and throat), or on particular techniques (like radiography or anaesthetics). This was orthodox medicine. Natural medicine, which until Virchow had been the only medicine (apart from surgery), was swept aside by the new technological generation, and its practitioners were ignored. It was a while before it began to make a comeback, but today more and more people are demanding to be treated the natural way and the old techniques are being revived and developed alongside the new.

It is interesting to think of this renaissance in the context of our cultural history. In the Renaissance of the eighteenth century, men cast their minds back to the past and gathered forgotten knowledge which enabled them to take a great step forward. Modern doctors of natural medicine are doing the same thing. Practitioners today are not cranks and quacks but serious men and women who combine modern techniques with the experience of generations, and the result is a whole new way of looking at medicine which shuns the synthetic and the unnatural.

### Where the orthodox and the unorthodox meet

The use of plants in healing has been shown to be the only concrete link between orthodox and natural medicine, being an intrinsic part of both traditional folk remedies and the international pharmaceutical market. This duality of purpose inevitably raises the questions: Can plants really work equally well in both spheres? When are they more effective? Are they ever harmful?

Just a step further and the entire relationship between the two medical schools is thrown into question. They seem to be poles apart. The whole of medicine is divided, creating a dilemma for the patient, whose one wish is to be healthy.

At this stage it is important to remember that in spite of their differences, from a scientific, humanitarian and historical point of view the two schools are united, and not divided. But this unity is born of necessity: disease must be conquered.

### Plants and herbs as remedies and stimulants

Plants have not only long been used by country people to cure and ward off all sorts of diseases in the absence of a doctor, but also to heighten the flavour of their cooking. Some plants, like thyme, are just as at home in the medicine chest as they are in the kitchen. Plants which are stimulants, like coffee, cocoa and tobacco, can also be put to both uses: the caffeine in black tea or coffee tastes good and heightens the senses; in aspirin, the same substance is used to contract the blood vessels and so help to relieve pain.

### What are drugs?

'Healing plants are those which contain substances beneficial to the health and which can be used wholly or in part for the purpose of healing.'

This definition neatly separates healing plants from all others, and especially from the weeds and herbs which are usually thrown into the cooking pot with them (metaphorically or otherwise).

In this book the term 'drug' is freely used alongside the concept of healing plants, even though today it has the most unpleasant associations. Recently there has been much talk of drug addicts, drug addiction and drug crimes, but it is only the misuse of drugs which has earned them their bad reputation and in medical circles the word is free of these ugly connotations.

The word 'drug' has its origins in an old Nordic word and means nothing more sinister than 'dried material'.

Today in plant medicine it is used to cover all sorts of dried plants and parts of plants, such as dried leaves, roots and blossoms.

## Healing agents

Not all parts of the same plant contain the same substances, so that you can find a plant whose leaves contain a healing agent but whose roots, for example, are medically worthless. This is why it is important to know more about healing agents and where to find them, so that the important parts of the plant are not discarded during collecting, and the useless ones not stored. A doctor will never prescribe a whole plant against a certain illness, but specify the part to be used. The season of the year and the manner in which the plants are prepared are also significant, as at certain times of the year a healing agent may be less powerful or found in less concentration in a particular plant. (More about this in the chapter on healing agents and how they work on page 23.)

Today there are two main types of healing agent. The pharmaceutical industry, which relies heavily on plants as well as on synthetic substances, markets a range of powerful 'specific' drugs, so called because they contain a single healing agent, derived either from chemicals or natural sources, and have been developed for one purpose only: to cure a specific disease. A specific drug would be used, for example, to cure a rare virus infection, and anyone not suffering from this virus would not benefit from taking the drug. These drugs obviously play an essential part in treating hospital patients who are suffering from serious illnesses or in an advanced stage of illness, but are far too drastic for the average person who pays a visit to the doctor because he simply doesn't feel well.

Any illness which is not severe should be treated not with a specific drug but with a 'general combination' drug. General combination drugs, as their names suggests, are delicately balanced preparations made from several substances, including catalysts, which work together in natural harmony.

Catalysts play an important role in all biological processes, and not least in healing. They stimulate, accelerate or control the chemical reaction between two or more substances without taking part in it themselves, thus moderating or heightening the powers of the healing agent.

Doctors in Middle European countries have always recognized the value of these milder, more natural general combination drugs, and they are now taking their rightful place in Western medicine alongside the stronger specific drugs.

## The long-term healing effects of plants

In many cases the immediate effects of healing plants are weak or even non-existent, and it can be quite a long time before they produce any results at all. This can be an advantage as well as a disadvantage: it's just a matter of letting nature take her course. But what does this mean in biological terms?

The majority of processes in a human or animal body are controlled by reflex actions, i.e. they are triggered off by an external stimulus and not by a voluntary decision. (Think of the doctor testing your reflexes by giving you a smart tap with a hammer just below the kneecap.) The kneecap reflex is not needed all the time, but other reflex muscles are in constant use, and are able to do without the external stimulus and work by themselves. These are the automatic reflexes and they control the body's muscles and all the inner organs, including the heart, the digestive system and the blood vessels, as well as co-ordinated activities like sitting, standing and walking. Whenever the sight of food makes your mouth water, the sight of someone you love makes your heart miss a beat or exertion makes it race, this is due to a muscle contraction activated by an automatic reflex.

Exactly the same processes have been observed taking place in the microscopic world of the cell. Automatic reflexes programme, control and co-ordinate all the body's activities, and without them life would not be possible.

But, as we have seen, all reflexes are first caused by stimulation, and when the stimulation is constant, the reflex becomes automatic. This works just as well if the stimulant is a chemical. The constant bombarding of a nerve fibre by a molecule will eventually produce an automatic reflex action, and it has been proved that this is how many medicines actually work. It also explains how people get addicted to drugs.

A specific drug, whether its base is chemical or herbal, will often take effect with only one dose and is very useful in the treatment of symptoms like pains, swellings or inflammations, which can be made to disappear overnight.

On the other hand, a general combination drug will have more than one function, consisting as it does of several substances which work together in natural harmony, perhaps none of which is strong enough to give immediate relief to a single pain or irrritation. However, taken over a period of time, general combination drugs will condition reflexes in the body which will produce effects comparable to those of specific drugs, without being as drastic. This is because they trigger off neuro-chemical reflexes which in time become automatic and continue even after the patient has stopped taking the drug. The advantage with this method is that the body brings about its own recovery and is unlikely to be vulnerable to the same complaint during or after convalescence.

Unlike specific drugs, which treat the symptoms, general combination drugs go right to the root of the disease and treat its cause. Casual therapy is an important principle of all natural medicine, including homoeopathy, radionics and hydrotherapy, and relies heavily on general stimuli to activiate the healing powers of the body by producing reflexes which eventually become automatic.

No-one would expect a lightning cure from a thermal bath: with this treatment as with any other natural therapy, nature must be allowed to take her course.

**Poisonous properties of healing plants**
Paracelsus, who was a pioneer of many branches of medicine, stated confidently that any medicine given in the wrong dose could be poisonous, and that the healing powers of a substance depended as much on quantity as on quality. Although Paracelsus had no means of scientifically checking his theory, modern technology has proved it to be correct: any healing agent has inherent poisonous properties which will be activated if it is given in the wrong dose. A medicine given in large quantities will react with the organism it enters and produce a poisonous, even deadly effect. Given in smaller quantities it can be beneficial; in smaller quantities still its effects will hardly be noticed.

**Finding the correct dose**
The greater the margin between a poisonous and a beneficial dose, the more useful a medicine will be. Thus the doctor will be able to prescribe a greater range of doses for a wider variety of ills without danger of harm. This factor is known to doctors as the 'therapeutic margin'. Substances with a low therapeutic margin have to be prescribed with extra care because only a small overdose would have harmful effects and might even cause death.

A good example of this is a poison called kurare (derived from a plant) used on the tips of arrows by South American Indians. Only a tiny quantity of this will paralyze and kill a man within seconds when applied to an open wound, yet a really minute amount of the same substance in the hands of an experienced anaesthetician can be used to relax muscles and prepare the body for a surgical operation. This is an instance of one drug with an extremely small therapeutic margin.

Unlike kurare, most drugs derived from plants have the advantage of a wide therapeutic margin, and in most cases the normal dosage can happily be doubled or trebled without causing any harmful side-effects. St John's wort, hops and valerian can all safely be taken as tranquillizers or soporifics in greatly increased doses. Because all these substances are natural and combine many individual elements working together in harmony, there is less danger of harm to the organism which absorbs them.

**Healing plants and the layman**
Even though natural drugs are potentially less harmful than chemical ones, there are those which must be treated with great care and understanding. One such is camomile, long prescribed by our grandmothers for all sorts of ills. Despite its harmless image, camomile can have very unpleasant effects when taken in too-large doses (see the entry on camomile on page 44). It is always essential to remember *to stick to the given dosage.* Do *not* think that because you feel that little bit less well, you should automatically give yourself a double dose of the recommended medicine, because it might

well do you harm instead of good. In such cases it is always imperative to consult a doctor or a pharmacist.

A further warning: some of the strongest drugs of all are derived from plants. One of them is kurare, but others hide behind more innocent exteriors. The foxglove, common in woodland clearings, the sweet-smelling lily of the valley, so popular with gardeners and the addictive drugs derived from hemp are far from being harmless. So when the doctor prescribes an exact dose of a drug which contains digitalis (derived from the foxglove), the patient must be sure not to increase it if he wants his condition to improve.

The purpose of this book, to encourage the use of plant remedies in the home, should not be taken by the reader as an unlimited licence for self-treatment. When in doubt, *always* consult your doctor or pharmacist.

However, all the plants and recipes described in this book have been especially chosen for use in the home, and are perfectly safe if the instructions are properly adhered to.

## When NOT to treat yourself

There are cases when the patient should definitely not treat himself, or should stop self-treatment straight away. In general, it is advisable to consult a doctor under the following circumstances:

1. If a complaint has persisted over a long period of time before treatment is considered.
2. If sudden drastic changes take place in the patient's condition, especially in the heart, circulation or breathing.
3. If the patient suffers continual or acute pain.
4. If the home-treatment is successful, but the patient returns to his previous condition after the treatment is left off.
5. If the home-treatment does not produce encouraging results within several days.

A doctor should in any case be called in to give advice on any long-term treatments. The symptoms of many serious illnesses do not seem serious in themselves, especially in the early stages, and it is often impossible for a layman to recognize what he is suffering from. In these cases too, a trained doctor will be able to diagnose a disease long before it has taken hold, and advise the patient on the best sort of treatment available.

These criteria apply not only to plant medicine but to any kind of treatment administered by someone who has not been fully trained in the subject. The greatest danger is perhaps that the layman can overlook or misinterpret the symptoms of serious diseases, which may become untreatable before they are recognized. It is always important to remember that what you neglect to do can be as decisive for your health as the treatment you take.

## Herbal versus orthodox medicine

Do herbal remedies have advantages over commercially produced medicines? This is not an easy question to answer. As we have seen many commercial medicines contain substances derived from plants as well as synthetic products, so it is first necessary to discount general combination drugs, which are phytotherapeutic in intent, and concentrate on their specific counterparts. It would not be fair in a book of this kind to dismiss specific drugs at one blow without considering the advantages they certainly do possess. There are of course cases in medicine where specific drugs are not only more effective but are the only possible method of treatment. All other remedies should be discarded in their favour. There is no doubt that the pharmaceutical industry and modern medical technology have combined to produce the most outstanding medical achievements, without which human lives would often be lost.

The following points are a useful guide as to when specific drugs should be employed:

1. In a matter of life and death the medicine with the most powerful immediate effect should obviously be preferred.
2. When the effects of all the available medicaments are weighed up and it becomes obvious that only a specific drug will be effective in curing the illness without causing undesirable side-effects.

In all cases the home doctor should remember one of the cast-iron rules of professional medicine: *nil nocere,* 'never do harm'. This precept must not be taken too literally (in the case of surgery, for example, the doctor often has to be cruel to be kind), but he should always work towards the better health of the patient even though an operation is sometimes unavoidable.

The patient's health is always the first aim of the doctor, and this is why even a doctor who is atuned to the advantages of natural medicine will prescribe a specific drug when he feels that a general combination drug or a purely phytotherapeutic remedy would be too weak or too slow to take effect. If a specific drug is the only treatment which will quickly and safely bring the patient back to health, then even the most enthusiastic doctor of natural medicine should not hesitate to prescribe it.

However, when it is a question of building up a patient's strength and getting him back into top form, the same doctor would no doubt advise a plant remedy such as can be found in this book. The natural harmonizing properties of plant remedies restore normal balance to the body's functions and allow it to build an invaluable immunity to disease. These remedies team up so well with other forms of natural treatment, that a doctor who is an expert on the subject might well recommend his patient to combine them with say, a course of thermal baths.

On balance then neither commercial drugs (whether plant- or synthetic-based), nor phytotherapeutic remedies should be used solely. They both have advantages and disadvantages, and they both have an essential role to play in modern medicine.

**Tolerance of drugs**
Why should it be true that both

humans and animals have a higher tolerance of plant remedies than they do of chemical drugs? One factor that should be taken into account is that the blood serum of almost all animal life has a remarkably similar constitution to that of seawater and of plant sap. All three contain much the same concentration of the most important ions, including sodium, potassium, calcium, magnesium and chlorine. Biological nihilists will call this pure chance, but it is a fact interesting enough to ponder over. The information we have suggests that pure plant remedies are more compatible with animal organisms than even general combination drugs. This would seem to suggest that all things in nature are balanced in a harmony which cannot easily be entered by anything that is artificially produced.

In the course of millions of years of evolution on this planet natural elements combined and recombined with each other until the perfect circumstances convened to produce the first forms of life. Each life-form contained natural substances specially adapted to react to the surroundings it was born in, and so a kind of symbiosis or interdependence developed between the organism and its environment. Each organism grew and changed to make the best use of the available supplies, so that a life-form which fed off one substance could live side by side with another organism to whom that substance was indigestible. (Horses are compatible with men in evolutionary terms because horses won't eat meat and men won't eat hay.)

The difference between the needs of one organism and those of the next creates no problem as long as there is enough nourishment to go round. Problems only occur when the natural balance between nourishment and growth is disturbed. A lack of food will result in malnutrition which leads to death. On the other hand, a superfluity of food will result in obesity which, if it does not cause death directly, at least hurries it on.

With these basic principles in mind and the knowledge that nourishment gives energy equals life, it is time to turn to the question of health.

## The healthy body

Health goes hand in hand with nourishment, energy and life, and there is no doubt that through the centuries of evolution on this planet health was achieved together with nourishment in the form of plants—man's first medicine.

Plants restored the balance of health to early man by providing his body with the organic substances it needed in times of sickness: when enough of the correct substances had been taken in, the patient returned to health. There were two pitfalls with this primitive healing plan:

1. If not enough of the right substances were available the illness continued.
2. If too much of the healing substance was taken the therapeutic margin would be passed and the patient would be poisoned and perhaps die.

Only when the right amount of the right substance was taken at the right time would the patient recover successfully.

The last 150 years have seen the production of many synthetic substances that never existed in nature. It can easily be imagined that when these man-made or artificial substances come into contact with an organism it has no means of assimilating them or making use of them to redress the balance of energy or health. It would also seem safe to assume, therefore, that quantities of the synthetic substances with which we bombard our bodies remain unchanged within us until our metabolism has learned how to react against them. This produces side-effects which appear so long after the original substance was taken that they are never associated with it.

This does not just apply to synthetic medicine either. Our bodies come into contact with many other artificial products each day: insecticides, detergents and preservatives in commercial foodstuffs are just a few of the offenders.

An example of an artificial substance taken as medicine and which builds up over the years inside the body is a mercury compound used to treat syphilis. A few decades ago syphilis was a very widespread disease and it was discovered that this compound was a better remedy than any other. Although its long-term effects on the body were not known, it was given to a great many people who found it highly successful.

Recently a doctor who runs a fasting clinic was supervising a group of middle-aged patients fasting to improve their health and rid their bodies of poisonous waste. Several days after the fast had begun the doctor noticed a distinct smell of mercury in the air and on questioning his patients he discovered to his astonishment that several of them had indeed been treated for syphilis with the well-known mercury compound in their youth. Their bodies had no means of dealing with the mercury, which had remained inside them for decades until it was flushed out by the purgative fasting process.

Obviously it is not possible to prove that natural medicines succeed where commercial drugs fail, and that after the healing process is completed they are eliminated from the body and not left behind to do untold slow damage. Nevertheless, it does seem likely that biological substances are more compatible with biological organisms than man-made substances, and that they would be more easily broken down, assimilated and disposed of than their synthetic counterparts. In any case, no doctor would deny that the more atuned a drug is to the biological processes of the body, the better its potential healing powers are.

### The body and nature
The body has an inbuilt compatibility with all natural organic substances, a compatibility which begins at birth and develops as the child grows to maturity. The relationship between man and nature is an important one,

and obviously vital for his survival in the modern world. To understand it fully, it is necessary to listen to the body's language and to meet its every need. Just as the night rider should trust his horse's sense of direction and not force him to go the way *he* thinks right, so anyone who is truly concerned about his health should not impose on his body any treatment which his instincts tell him is wrong.

Our children often show us the way in this respect, for after all they are closer to nature than their parents. When children persistently dislike a particular kind of food, it is almost always for a good biological reason. Parents often find it difficult to accept this and tend to force their sons and daughters to eat up food which actually disagrees with them on the pretext that they are being merely disobedient. Telling a child to 'eat up or else' is certainly not going to encourage harmonious relations between the child's body and the rest of nature.

People refuse certain foods because they know instinctively that they are not good for them, so it is hardly surprising that medicines which suit some people disagree with others. It is always wise to make a note of your reactions to different drugs and tell your doctor of them, so that he has some guide as to your tolerance and a better chance of prescribing a suitable medicine the first time around.

The aim of every therapeutic treatment is to establish and maintain a state of harmony and balance between the patient and his environment. The most frequent disruptions of this balance are only minor irritations which can easily be levelled out or compensated for with gentle natural therapy carried out at home. Simple preparations like camomile tea or tincture of valerian can be just what is needed when you feel under the weather, and with this book as a guide, plant remedies will become a valuable part of your programme for natural health.

# CHAPTER TWO

# HEALING AGENTS AND HOW THEY WORK

There are two main types of substance formed in healing plants during the course of their natural metabolic processes, and both have an important medical role. The healing agents themselves are the active substances; the inactive, or ballast substances determine how effective they will be by making the body more, or less receptive to their powers.

Most healing plants contain several pharmacologically active substances, one of which will be dominant, and it is this substance which influences the choice of plant by the phytotherapist. But the importance of the secondary healing agents should not be underestimated, because without them the primary agent could have a totally different effect: it is the natural combination of active and ballast substances rather than the working of a single agent which puts the body back on the road to health.

The variety of healing substances in a plant should be known to the collector, as should be the equally important fact that they can be found in different quantities in different parts of the plant. Sometimes the most valuable part of the plant is its blossom, at other it may be leaves, roots, seeds, fruit, or even bark.

Another fact worth knowing is that the potency of healing plants varies with the seasons and that some are always far more powerful than others, and so should not be used in home medicine. However, *most* healing plants can be used safely at home, as long as you know the correct season for harvesting and the best way of preparing the medicine to guard against harmful effects. The correct method of storing plants ensures that they lose little of their potency and this is essential because some treatments take up to eight weeks to complete.

The word 'drug', as stated in the introduction of this book, has been used reputably in medicine for centuries and is synonymous with the term 'healing agent', just as the word 'druggist' is synonymous with the word 'chemist'. No-one using this book should be afraid of becoming addicted to any of the drugs described in it: they are not that kind of drug.

In order to know more about the use of plants in home medicine it is first necessary to get a basic grasp of some of the healing agents they contain.

### Alkaloid drugs

These are mostly very potent substances and taken in overdose they can have poisonous effects. This makes them unsuitable for use in teas and infusions, though they are widely used by the pharmaceutical industry. They include atropine, a poison found in deadly nightshade, morphine, from the opium poppy, or colchicine from the autumn crocus. Caffein and theobromide in coffee, black tea and cocoa are also alkaloids, and so these beverages should not be drunk in large quantities. However, alkaloids are also sometimes present in reduced quantities in plants not usually regarded as containing any poisonous substances. Their function here is to act as a catalyst to the healing process without being involved in it directly themselves.

### Bitter drugs

There are a great number of healing plants that taste bitter, but the term 'bitter drugs' refers solely to those plants which contain a healing agent whose potency is due to its bitter qualities.

In phytotherapy bitter drugs are known as *amara*. They can be subdivided into the following groups:

1. Pure bitters, *amara tonica.*
2. Bitter drugs which contain a significant quantity of essential oil and hence taste bitter and aromatic, *amara aromatica.*
3. *Amara acria,* which taste acid and sharp.

Although many healing plants can be classified as *amara,* phytotherapists have been able to whittle this number down and select a more manageable group of plants which can be especially recommended for their excellent healing effects. This makes it easier for the layman, who is not obliged to learn about the whole range of *amara.*

The secretion of the digestive juices in the stomach is controlled by bitters, and this is one area where they can be said to have a beneficial effect. Bitter drugs are therefore highly recommended in cases of loss of appetite and indigestion. They are equally good at strengthening the body when it has been weakened by ill health and can be of great help to convalescents or those suffering from anaemia or nervous exhaustion. Even patients with chronic gastritis can be treated with infusions of lesser centaury and wormwood, both of which are bitter drugs.

*Amara aromatica,* which contain essential oils as well as bitters, differ from the pure *amara* only in that the presence of the essential oils makes them more widely applicable. Mugwort, wormwood, angelica, St Benedict's herb and sweet flag are important members of this group. They are effective not only in the stomach but also in the intestine, gall bladder and liver. Because essential oils are antiseptic, *amara aromatica* can protect these areas against bacteria and parasites and are particularly highly valued in the treatment of zymosis. Some of these drugs have a slightly diuretic side-effect which can be most welcome. As expectorants (in the treatment of coughs and inflamed throats) they are slightly less useful.

*Amara acria* are very rare amongst native plants, being more common in exotics such as pepper and ginger. The sharpness of these drugs aids the circulation besides improving the digestion like the other *amara*. Indeed it has been found that bad digestion hinders the circulation more than was previously realized, and *amara, amara aromatica* and *amara acris* are all effective in treating this complaint.

## Essential oils as healing agents

Essential oils are constituents of plants which have a strong, but almost always pleasant smell. Although they evaporate easily they hardly ever dissolve in water. There are hardly any plants which contain no essential oils at all, but those used in phytotherapy contain a particularly high concentration of these fragrant oils. Two of the most prominent botanical families of plants to fall into this area are the labiates and umbelliferae. Here, as in other plants, the essential oils are stored in special receptacles which may take the form of cells or ducts.

Essential oils are composed of a variety of different substances, and up to fifty can be identified in a single type of oil. These substances can help to relieve light or severe irritation of the skin, they can act as expectorants in the treatment of coughs, they can be diuretics, relieve cramp and act as tonics to strengthen the stomach, intestines, gall bladder and liver. They are also used to treat infectious diseases and can help rid the body of bacteria and even viruses, although it must not be assumed that they will necessarily completely kill them. For further details see Chapter 4.

## Tannin as a healing agent

Tannin is a botanical agent which is capable of binding albumen in the skin and the mucous membrane to form an insoluble protective layer resistant to disease. Herein lies its healing power, because it can separate the bacteria which have settled on the skin and the mucous membrane from their source of nutrition. Tannin can be the primary healing agent in a plant (e.g. tormentil, oak bark, blueberry etc.), it can act as a catalyst, and in some cases it can even have a harmful effect and irritate the stomach wall. A way round this is to prepare a cold infusion of the plant prescribed so that only a small proportion of the tannin is absorbed.

Drugs containing tannin are useful to gargle with if the patient is suffering from a sore throat, as a mouthwash against inflamed gums, in the form of a compress to heal open wounds, and especially as a treatment against diarrhoea. In hot water they can effectively be used to bathe haemorrhoids, bunions and general inflammations of the skin.

## Glycoside drugs as healing agents

Glycosides are very common substances in the plant world. Their powers are so many and varied that their name alone tells very little of their effectiveness as healing agents. To check on their individual properties, see Chapter 4. However, all glycosides do have one factor in common. They can be separated by hydrolysis (a process in which a substance divides as it absorbs water) into a sugar and a non-sugar (aglycone). Aglycone is the substance which by and large is responsible for the healing effect of the plant which contains it. It is the aglycone in the foxglove (digitalis) which is valued in the treatment of heart disease; other aglycones are to be found in the bark of the alder buckthorn, the root of the primrose and the leaves of the bearberry. The effect of many acidic drugs can also be traced back to aglycones.

## Drugs containing silicic acid

Plants from the families of horsetail, borage and grass absorb silicic acid from the ground and store it in the cell membranes or in the protoplasma. In many cases the salts contained in silicic acid (silicates) will dissolve in water. Silicic acid is indispensable to the human body (especially to the connective tissue, the skin, hair and nails), and a silicate deficiency in the diet can be made up for by taking drugs containing silicic acid. One of the drugs most often used in pharmaceutics to this end is the field horsetail, which can be taken in infusion or applied externally as a gargle, mouthwash or bath.

## Mucilaginous drugs

'Mucilage' in the botanical and pharmacological sense refers to carboniferous substances which swell when water is added to them to form a viscous fluid. Mucilaginous drugs are widespread throughout the plant kingdom, but only a few plants contain them in great enough quantities to make them useful to medicine (e.g. marsh mallow, Icelandic moss and flax). In the majority of cases, however, they do intensify the effect of other healing agents present in the plants, especially in the relief of irritations.

The mucilage forms a fine layer on the surface of the mucous membrane, protects it from irritants and rapidly soothes existing inflammations. Because mucilage is not absorbed, its effects are always purely local. It will therefore only relieve coughs caused directly by irritations in the mouth and throat. Mucilaginous drugs have a slightly laxative effect because they loosen the contents of the bowel and absorb water from them (see linseed page 61). One of their side-effects is to weaken the sensibility of taste, especially for sour or acidic food and drink. An interesting example is that although raspberries contain less sugar and more acid than redcurrants, they are richer in mucilage and therefore taste sweeter.

## Vitamins, minerals and trace elements

Any list of the properties of plants should include the so-called 'essential elements'. They are necessary to every organism to build its framework, of connective tissue, bones and teeth, and to provide its cell structure. They form the foundation of the enzymes and hormones, activate the metabolism and the body's organs and control the urinary tract.

Without these substances no form of life could exist, and so of course it is essential that we take them in with our food and drink. There are lots of nutrients to be found in plants, like vegetables, salads and fruit, and in the treatment of disease, which is after all caused by a lack of these substances, it is only natural to seek out those plants which contain especially large quantities of nutrients.

Some of the necessary minerals, vitamins and trace elements are soluble and can be taken as infusions. Some plants are especially useful for their vitamin content, for example the rose hip (see page 51).

# CHAPTER THREE

# THE ANATOMY OF PLANTS

It is important for anyone who is interested in the healing power of plants to know something about their structure, about their different organs and how they work.

Each part of the plant plays a role in its most important function: propagation. The root nourishes the shoots, leaves and flowers, and gives the plant the strength to reproduce via its fruit. Normally, roots are underground organs which anchor the plant in position in the soil, and the shoots, leaves and flowers grow above ground. There are of course exceptions to this rule (see page 30 figure 4).

*The root* draws moisture and nourishment in solution from the soil and anchors the plant in position. There are various kinds of root:

1. The tap-root grows vertically into the soil and sends off weaker shoots to either side.
2. Carrots and beets are examples of thicker tap-roots grown as food for man and fodder for animals.

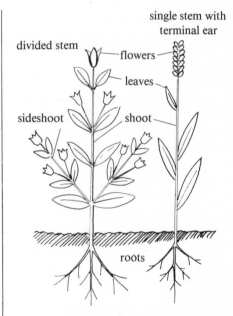

Figure 1. The basic plant

3. Fibrous roots form an underground network of equally strong roots.

*The shoot* can be divided into two categories: the green stalk, and the woody stem. Green stalks are pro-

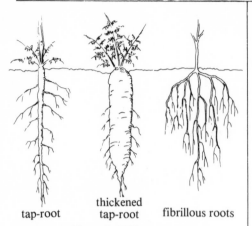

tap-root    thickened    fibrillous roots
            tap-root

Figure 2. Different roots

The leaves grow from the shoot, and in the axes of these leaves, side-shoots develop and grow other leaves. Flowers can also grow in clusters or singly from the axes, either directly or on stalks.

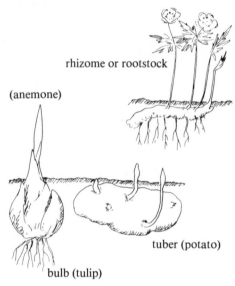

rhizome or rootstock

(anemone)

tuber (potato)

bulb (tulip)

Figure 4. Underground shoots

duced by annual plants, those which complete their life cycle in one year, germinating in spring and dying down in autumn, and by biennials, plants which take two years to complete their life cycle. Perennials, those which live for more than two years, also have green stalks, though sometimes they develop the woody stems character-istic of trees and shrubs, which are usually the most long-lived plants.

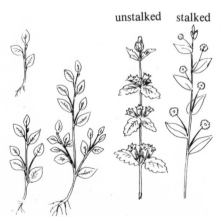

unstalked    stalked

Figure 3. Development of the leaves
and sideshoots

Shoots aren't always formed above the surface of the earth: sometimes they grow below it from a root which stores the food they need to survive. A rhizome or rootstock like the anemone is one such which creeps and spreads horizontally just below the earth's surface. Another is the onion-like bulb characteristics of the tulip, which is made of layers of fleshy underground leaves. A third is the tuber, and an example of this is the common potato.

Shoots or stalks which grow above ground can be round (in cross-section), two-cornered, square, triangular or ribbed.

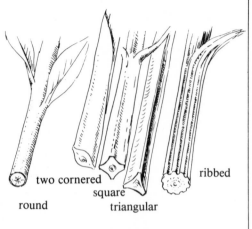

Figure 5. Shoots and stalks

*The leaves* assimilate organic substances necessary for the nutrition of the plant. They take in various sugars and starches from rainwater and carbon dioxide from the air. This process is called photosynthesis and involves chlorophyll, the green colouring substance present in all plants, interacting with energy from the sun. The leaves are green because they are full of chlorophyll, and they are flat so that they have the maximum surface area exposed to the elements which give them life: air, rain and sun. They grow from their stalks in various formations: in rosettes around the stalk; in opposite pairs at right-angles to each other along the stalk; in opposite pairs parallel to each other, and alternately along the stalk.

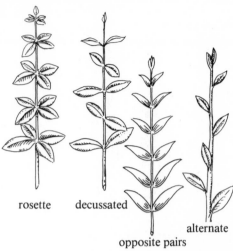

Figure 6. How leaves form on the stem

The stalk of a leaf can be anything from very long to non-existent and sometimes the stalk even grows through the leaf. The leafblade itself can also be very varied. For the identification of a leaf its edge and the way its veins divide it up are as important as its shape.

Leaves can grow directly onto the stem (the stem sometimes even grows through the leaves) or be attached to it by a stalk.

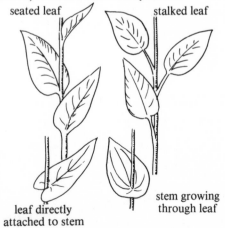

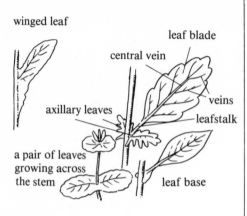

winged leaf

leaf blade

central vein

axillary leaves

veins

leafstalk

a pair of leaves
growing across
the stem

leaf base

Figure 7. Leaf information

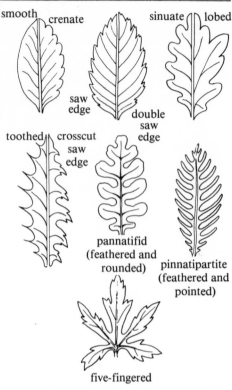

smooth   crenate                    sinuate   lobed

saw
edge                        double
                            saw
toothed   crosscut           edge
          saw
          edge

pannatifid
(feathered and
rounded)      pinnatipartite
              (feathered and
                  pointed)

five-fingered

Figure 9. Edges of simple leaves

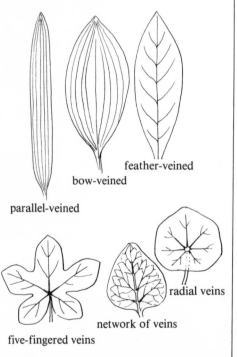

feather-veined

bow-veined

parallel-veined

radial veins

network of veins

five-fingered veins

Figure 8. Leafblades and veins

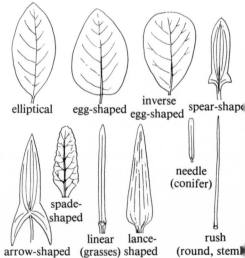

elliptical   egg-shaped   inverse   spear-shape
                          egg-shaped

needle
(conifer)

spade-
shaped

arrow-shaped   linear   lance-   rush
               (grasses) shaped   (round, stem)

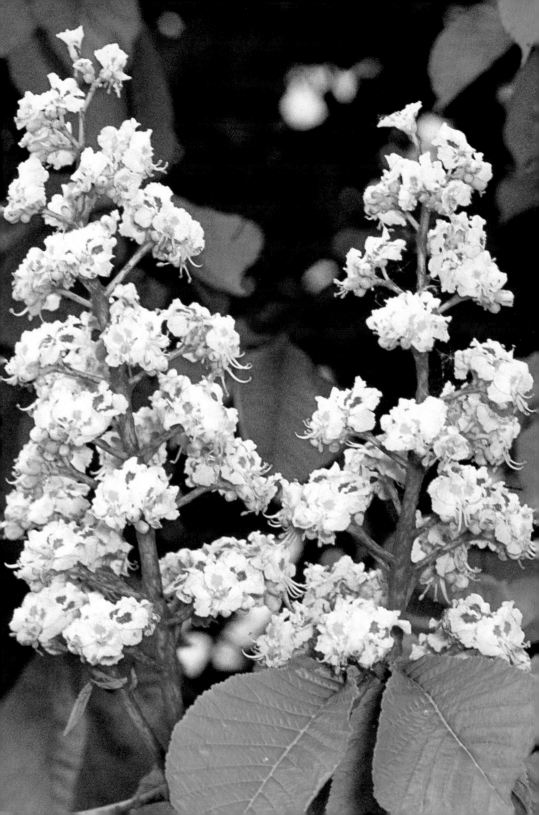

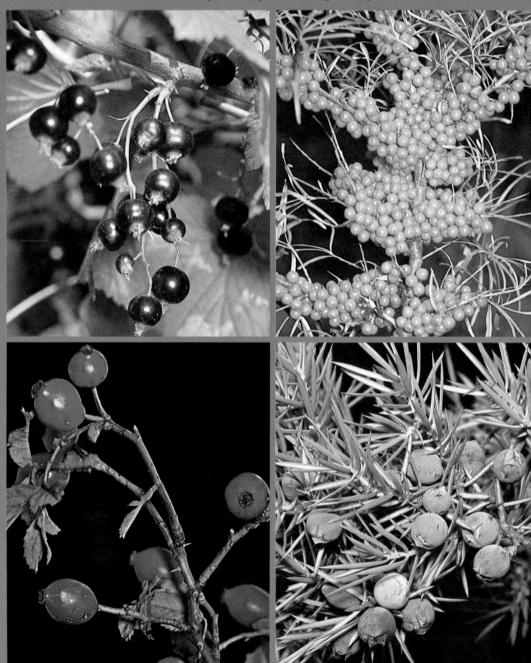

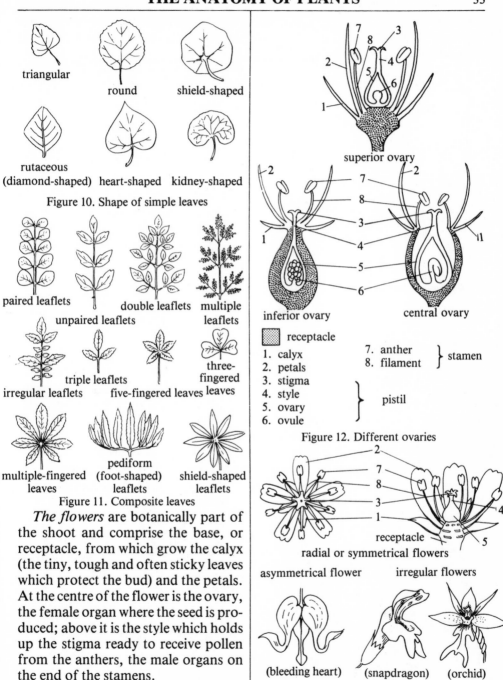

triangular

round

shield-shaped

rutaceous
(diamond-shaped)   heart-shaped   kidney-shaped

Figure 10. Shape of simple leaves

paired leaflets

unpaired leaflets

double leaflets   multiple
leaflets

irregular leaflets

triple leaflets

five-fingered leaves

three-
fingered
leaves

multiple-fingered
leaves

pediform
(foot-shaped)
leaflets

shield-shaped
leaflets

Figure 11. Composite leaves

superior ovary

inferior ovary

central ovary

receptacle

1. calyx
2. petals
3. stigma
4. style
5. ovary
6. ovule

7. anther
8. filament } stamen

} pistil

Figure 12. Different ovaries

receptacle

radial or symmetrical flowers

asymmetrical flower

irregular flowers

(bleeding heart)   (snapdragon)   (orchid)

Figure 13. Flower forms

*The flowers* are botanically part of the shoot and comprise the base, or receptacle, from which grow the calyx (the tiny, tough and often sticky leaves which protect the bud) and the petals. At the centre of the flower is the ovary, the female organ where the seed is produced; above it is the style which holds up the stigma ready to receive pollen from the anthers, the male organs on the end of the stamens.

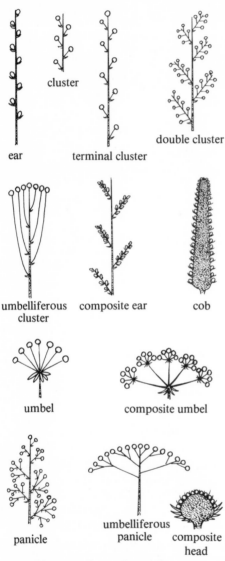

cluster

double cluster

ear    terminal cluster

umbelliferous    composite ear    cob
cluster

umbel    composite umbel

panicle    umbelliferous    composite
panicle    head

Figure 14. Formation of flowers

Only in rare cases like the tulip does the plant produce one single flower, and mostly several blooms are produced together in a cluster, an ear, an umbel or a panicle.

*The fruit* is formed after the flowers have been fertilized by the pollen and died down, leaving the seeds to ripen inside the ovary walls, which can take several forms:

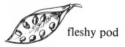

fleshy pod

1. Fleshy pod. The ovary forms two elongated 'leaves' which house the seeds. When they are ripe it splits at the outer seam to release them.

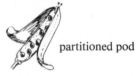

partitioned pod

2. Partitioned pod. This is similar to the above, except that the seeds are attached not to the pod wall, but to a thin skin which divides the two 'leaves'. When the seeds are ripe the 'leaves' spring apart rolling upwards from the partition and release them.

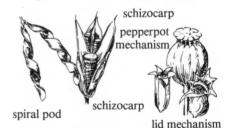

schizocarp

pepperpot mechanism

spiral pod    schizocarp

lid mechanism

Figure 15. Seeds

3. The spiral pod. In this case, the 'leaves' split apart and twist as they dry, dispersing the seeds in all directions.

4. The capsule. This is rounder and plumper than the pod. There are three types:

   a) the schizocarp, which splits in one or more places horizontally to free the seeds;

   b) the lid mechanism which opens at the top; and

   c) the pepperpot mechanism which shakes out seeds from holes under the 'lid'.

These are all forms of fruit, though the word itself more often conjures up something edible. A berry is a wholly fleshy fruit; a nut has a hard shell which contains a seed, and a stone fruit (or drupe) has a fleshy outer layer which conceals a stone or kernel. A multiple fruit consists of tiny nuts which sit on a fleshy core or receptacle. An example of this is the strawberry. Blackberries are similar, but their seeds are stones and not nuts.

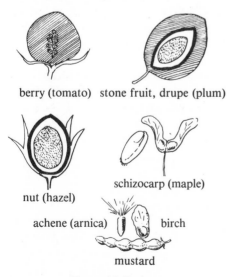

Figure 16. Fruits

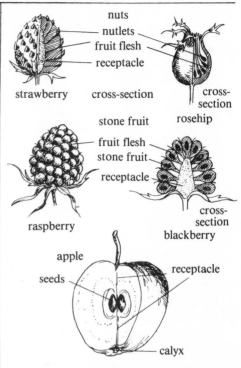

Figure 17. Edible fruits or pseudocarps

## General rules for collecting and drying healing plants

The prime requisites in collecting healing plants are to be quite sure that your identification of such plants is correct, and to learn which parts of a given plant are medically useful. Some plants are posionous and represent a real danger to the ill-informed through misidentification. Here are some other rules which should always be observed:

1. Never harvest your plants in rain, mist or damp weather. The best time of the day for harvesting is in the early morning, but you should make sure that the plants are free of dew.

2. Only plants which are quite clean should be harvested. Dirt or dust makes them worthless, as you should not wash them before use. Make sure that the soil in which the plants are growing is not polluted, and do not pick from plants growing by busy roadsides where they may be affected by the lead from exhaust fumes.

3. The leaves should be plucked when still quite young, but must be fully developed. The flowers should be in full bloom, but still young and fresh.

4. If you are harvesting the whole plant, then it should be gathered when it is just coming into bloom. Do acquaint yourself, though, with the Conservation of Wild Plants Act which prohibits the culling of rootstocks and rare plants.

5. Collect fruit only when they are fully ripe.

6. Collect only the roots that are strong and fully developed. This applies to rootstocks (rhizomes) as well.

It is necessary to dry plants and plant material before it is put to medical use to stop the natural fermentation that would otherwise occur. The drying process also ensures that fungi and bacteria are killed off. Drying is a way of preserving the healing agents in the plant and it should take place as soon after they are harvested as possible. The ideal conditions for drying plants are cool, shady and airy. Bright sunlight will often dry out important oils contained in the leaves, flowers and fruits. The best way to dry your harvest is to spread it out thinly on a sieve or finely meshed cooling tray and leave it in a cool airy place. If you are drying the whole plant, it is often convenient to hang it up in a bunch from the ceiling.

Plants can be dried successfully in artificial heat, provided the temperature is right. All plants and parts of plants which are aromatic contain essential oils, and these should be dried at a temperature of 35°C (95°F), whereas other plants which do not contain oils can safely stand 60°C (140°F). However, with all plants you should remember to keep the air fresh and circulating well in order to avoid fermentation.

Roots and rhizomes should be cut in half lengthways, unless they are fine or fibrillated, and tubers should be sliced.

Once your harvest has dried out, it should be stored in air-tight jars.

## THE COLLECTOR'S CALENDAR

| Plant | Page | Location | Part Used | Harvest Time |
|---|---|---|---|---|
| Aniseed | 39 | wild in overgrown gardens (not in UK) | dried fruit | Jul-Sep |
| Arnica | 40 | poor soil in mountainous regions; turfy flatlands (not in UK) | flowers | Jun-Jul |
| Balm | 41 | cultivated in gardens | leaves | Jul-Aug |
| Bearberry | 42 | moorland and heathland | leaves | May-Jun and autumn |
| Bilberry | 43 | sparse woodland; marshland | ripe fruit | Jul-Sep |
| Buckthorn (Alder) | 43 | mountain pasture; marshland; hedges | bark | Apr-Jun |
| Camomile | 44 | verges; cornfields; fallow land | flowers | May-Jul |
| Caraway | 46 | wild in overgrown gardens (not in UK) | dried fruit | Jul-Sep |
| Coltsfoot | 47 | in most clay or loam at the edges of woods; railway embankments; riversides | young leaves | Apr-Jul |
| Comfrey | 49 | damp meadows, ditches | root | Apr-May |
| Cowslip | 49 | meadowland; woodland | root and flowers | Apr-May |
| Dandelion | 50 | meadows; fields; gardens; wasteland | root and plant | May-Sep |
| Dog rose (rosehip) | 51 | hedges; sunny banks | ripe fruit | Sep-Oct |
| Eyebright | 52 | dry pastureland; cliffs; sparse woodland | whole plant | Jul-Sep |
| Elder | 60 | hedgerows | flowers | May-Jun |
| Fennel | 53 | wild in overgrown gardens | dried fruit | Jul-Sep |

| Plant | Page | Location | Part Used | Harvest Time |
|---|---|---|---|---|
| Field Horsetail | 54 | ditches; woodland; wasteland; loamy fields | summer shoots or 'horsetails' | May-Jul |
| Gentian | 55 | European mountain pasture-land; cultivated | root | Sep-Oct |
| Greater Celandine | 56 | gardens; waste ground | whole plant | Apr-Aug root in Sep-Oct |
| Hawthorn | 57 | hedges | flowers | May-Jun |
| Heartsease | 58 | meadowland; gardens | whole plant | Jul-Aug |
| Juniper | 51 | heathland; sparse woodland | berries | Oct-Nov |
| Lesser Centaury | 46 | sparse woodland; damp meadowland | whole plant | Jun-Aug |
| Lime | 59 | parks; gardens; woods | flowers | Jun-Jul |
| Milk Thistle | 61 | wild or cultivated in gardens | fruit | Sep |
| Peppermint | 63 | cultivated in gardens | leaves | Jul-Aug |
| St John's Wort | 64 | woods; sunny hillsides; dry fields; verges | whole plant | Jun-Aug |
| Sweet Flag | 65 | river banks | rhizome | Jun-Jul |
| Tormentil | 66 | woodlands; meadows; moorland | root | Jul-Aug |
| Valerian | 67 | damp pastureland; river banks; damp woodland | rhizome | Sep-Oct |
| Wormwood | 68 | stoney, uncultivated ground; rubbish tips | upper stem with flowers | Jun-Aug |
| Yarrow | 69 | dry fields; verges; cattle tracks | whole plant | Jun-Sep |

# CHAPTER FOUR

# A CATALOGUE OF HEALING PLANTS

## ANISEED

*Pimpinella
anisum*

Family:
Umbelliferae

**Part used:** Dried fruit (*Fructus anisi vulgaris*).

**Helps:** Wind, stomach cramps and coughs.

**Description:** This plant, known for the culinary and medicinal use of its seeds, was originally grown only in the orient, but today it is cultivated extensively in Europe. It is an umbelliferous plant, growing up to two feet (half a metre) high. Its roots are spindly and its lower leaves are stalked and roundish in shape with toothed edges. Higher up the stalk the leaves divide into three lobes, and the uppermost leaves are distinctly feathery. The fruits are round and give off a strong aroma due to the essential oils they contain. These oils consist of 80 to 90 per cent anethole.

**Active contents:** Anise has a great deal in common with fennel (see page 53) and caraway (see page 46). All three are used in cooking as well as in medicine, and all belong to the Umbelliferae family. The fruits of cultivated plants are to be preferred to those gathered in the wild because they are more aromatic. Each contains an essential oil suitable for treating wind and stomach upsets, as well as acting as an expectorant (it soothes irritations of the mucous membrane and is thus useful in treating coughs).

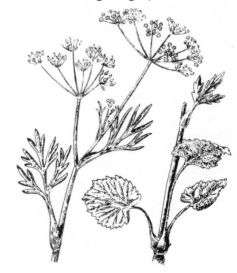

There are many healing plants which have a beneficial effect on the stomach and digestive tract, but aniseed, caraway and fennel are most often used in the treatment of chronic wind.
**To prepare the tea:** Pour boiling water into a cup over one teaspoonful of crushed seeds and strain after leaving for ten minutes. Aniseed and fennel teas are to be preferred to caraway, especially in the case of small children, as the taste is more pleasant. However, a mixture of all three is highly recommended. Using equal parts of aniseed, fennel and caraway, make up an ounce (25g) tea mixture. To make the drink put one teaspoonful of the tea in a cup and pour over boiling water. Allow to draw, covered, for twenty minutes before straining. Take one cupful three times a day after meals.

## ARNICA

*Arnica*             Family:
*montana*       Compositae

**Part used:** Flowers (*Flos arnicae*).
**Helps:** Cuts, grazes, sprains, bruises, bleeding and open wounds when applied externally. As a mouthwash it soothes inflammations of the mouth and throat; and taken internally it calms palpitations of the heart, but seek expert advice before using.
**Description:** Arnica is a mountain plant which grows best in European mountain pastureland or heathland, but it can also be found in the lowlands where it prefers the springy turf of sandy grassland. At the base of its tough green stalk, which can grow to a height of 20 inches (50cm), is a rosette

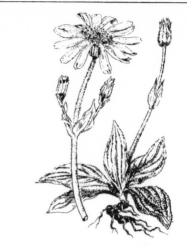

of leaves. One or two pairs of smaller leaves grow from the stalk, and from these spring secondary flower heads, the main one being at the top of the stem. The yellow blooms grow from a hairy calyx, and their petals each have three 'teeth'. This is important when identifying the plant.
**Harvesting tips:** Arnica flowers are ready for picking in June and July and they should be dried immediately if they are not to be used fresh(as in tincture or spirit of arnica). Tincture of arnica is used in preference to a tea. Unfortunately arnica does not grow in England, but in Southern Germany, where it is a common plant, it is to be found in every home medicine chest.
**Active contents:** Arnica contains essential oils, bitter matter, tannin and two flavone-glycosides (astragallin and isoquerzetin). The effectiveness of the drug is usually attributed to these glycosides alone, but it must be remembered that it is the combined action of all the elements in a plant that makes it medically useful.

**To prepare the tincture:** Mix dried arnica flowers with 70 per cent alcohol in the ratio of 1:10. If using fresh flowers use alcohol and flowers in equal amounts. After about fourteen days, strain through a muslin cloth, pressing out as much liquid as you can. Leave for two days to settle, then filter off any sediment before using.

To dilute the tincture mix a dessert-spoonful of tincture with half a pint (¼ litre). Such a dilution will be found to be more effective in compresses than using the tincture neat.

To make a mouthwash stir a tea-spoonful of tincture into a glass of water. Gargle and rinse round the mouth, then spit out.

Arnica can also be used internally to help the circulation but care should be taken and expert advice is best sought. The suggested dosage is ten to fifteen drops of the tincture three times a day. A good way to take them is on a cube of sugar.

**To prepare arnica tea:** Arnica tea can be used instead of the tincture and should be drunk in small sips for the best calming effect. Boil up one or two teaspoonsful of dried arnica flowers in half a pint (¼ litre) water and strain after ten minutes.

## BALM

*Melissa officinalis*

Family: Labiatae

**Part used:** Leaves (*Folia melissae*).
**Helps:** Nervous stomach upsets, 'flu and colds, insomnia.
**Description:** Balm originated in the eastern Mediterranean and, although

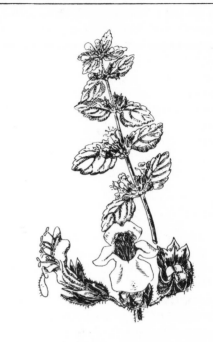

not often found growing wild in England, it is cultivated as a garden plant and has become quite popular in the herb garden, and rightly so, for apart from its medical usefulness it has an excellent flavour. It is an ancient plant, much used and highly thought of in traditional medicine. It grows to about two feet (60cm) in height and its leaves are lemon scented.

**Harvesting tips:** The leaves must be collected before the plant blooms because when balm is in flower its leaves don't taste or smell as pleasant.
**Active contents:** Fresh balm contains a small percentage of essential oil as well as tannin and bitter matter. It is a gentle tranquillizer which makes it a good remedy for anyone of a nervous disposition, or someone unable to sleep at night.

**To prepare balm tea:** Take two tea-spoonsful of chopped balm leaves per cup and pour on boiling water. Cover and allow the tea to brew for ten minutes. The tranquillizing effect of balm is also useful in the treatment of nervous stomach upsets because, apart from being a sedative, balm can relieve cramps and cure flatulance.

## BEARBERRY

*Arctostaphylos*                Family:
*uva ursi*                          Ericaceae

**Part used:** Leaves (*Folia uvae-ursi*).
**Helps:** Bladder and kidney trouble, and acts as a disinfectant to the urethra.
**Description:** The bearberry belongs to the heather family, and is to be found mainly on moor and heathland. Its leaves are leathery, its flowers pink, and in autumn it bears red berries.
**Harvesting tips:** The medically useful part of this plant is its leaves, which preferably should be collected in autumn when they are at their most potent.
**Active contents:** The glycoside arbutin is the most important active substance in the leaves of the bearberry. Arbutin only works in the medium of non-acidic urine, so it is important to avoid acids in the diet when undergoing a bearberry tea treatment. Cut out sour things such as fruit juice and vinegar. There is also a lot of tannin in bearberry leaves.
**To prepare bearberry tea:** Formerly it was believed that the leathery leaves of the bearberry had to be boiled for a long time before their potency would

be released, but this method produced tea so unpleasant that many patients were unable to continue the treatment through stomach upsets. It is now known that prolonged boiling releases a large quantity of tannin from the leaves, and a better method is to steep the leaves in cold water for twelve to twenty-four hours. This will be sufficient to activate the arbutin without spoiling the taste of the tea.

Strain and heat the liquid before drinking. One cup two to three times a day should be sufficient. The tea is to be highly recommended for inflammation of the bladder caused by chills and colds. However, should the inflammation continue without improvement for longer than a week it is advisable to visit your doctor. It is, in any case, wise to consult him before

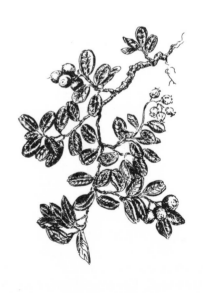

beginning any treatment of this nature, because often serious kidney illnesses which cannot be cured by plant medicine alone can be mistaken for minor complaints of the bladder.

## BILBERRY

*Vaccinium* Family:
*myrtillus* Vacciniaceae

**Part used:** Ripe fruits (*Fructus myrtilli*).
**Helps:** Diarrhoea; and can be used as a gargle for inflammation of the mouth and throat.
**Description:** The bilberry (or blueberry) is a straggly bush which grows as ground cover up to about a foot (30cm) high and is found especially in woodland areas and marshland. Its berries are blue-black and often partially hidden under its sparse dark green leaves. When squashed the berries leave a reddish stain and they were once used as a dye.

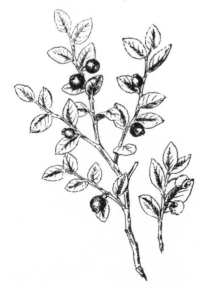

**Active contents:** The bilberry is an excellent source of tannin (the dried fruit contains about 7 per cent) and the colouring agent in the fruit is believed to have an anti-bacterial quality.

Although fresh bilberries contain plenty of vitamins (A, B-complex and C) and minerals (manganese and potassium) and are as delicious as they are nutritious, they have little or no effect on diarrhoea and should be taken as a medicine only when they are dry.

Dried bilberries can be taken as they are, but it is better to prepare a concentrated solution of the fruit juice and drink a small wineglassful as required.
**To prepare bilberry tea:** Pour a pint (½ litre) of cold water over three dessertspoonsful of dried berries and boil for ten minutes. Strain and cool and the tea will be ready to drink. For the best effects drink a glass of tea several times a day, and if you are suffering from diarrhoea an improvement will soon be noticed. It also makes a useful gargle to relieve inflammation of the mouth, throat and gums.

Another useful plant which works equally well against diarrhoea is Hare's Foot Clover (*Trifolium arvense*).

## BUCKTHORN, ALDER

*Rhamnus* Family:
*frangula* Rhamnaceae

**Part used:** Bark (*Cortex frangulae*).
**Helps:** Constipation.
**Description:** The alder buckthorn is a tall shrub frequently found on hillsides, in copses and in hedgerows. It grows up to 20 feet (6m) high and is

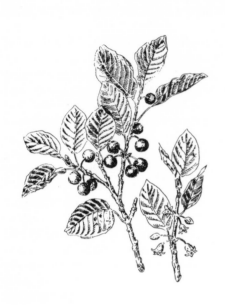

recognized by the large number of grey-white pores which speckle its otherwise smooth and gleaming grey-brown bark. The flowers are small and unremarkable and grow in groups of two to six from the base of the leaves. After they have been fertilized they develop into green, then red, and finally blue-black (or almost purple) stoned fruits. The leaves grow alternately, are elliptical, smooth-edged, and have a shiny upper surface.

**Harvesting tips:** The bark of the alder buckthorn is easily collected and dried, but *it must be stored for at least a year before use.* If the bark is used fresh it will irritate the stomach and cause vomiting.

**Active contents:** The alder buckthorn contains anthroquimone glycoside drugs which are also found in senna

leaves, aloes and some types of rhubarb. It is milder than aloes or senna and slightly more efficient than rhubarb.

**To prepare alder buckthorn tea:** Soak a teaspoonful of chopped bark (at least one year old) in a cupful of cold water for twelve hours with or without boiling first. Although often taken on its own, it is a good idea to combine it with something like aniseed to get rid of wind.

## CAMOMILE

*Matricaria*          Family:
*chamomilla*          Compositae

**Part used:** Flowers (*Flos chamomillae vulgaris*).

**Helps:** Complaints of the stomach and intestines and any sort of inflammation, particularly that of the mouth and throat. It is also good for wounds that are slow to heal.

**Description:** Camomile is an unfussy plant, having no preference for any particular soil type or position. It is native to most countries in northern Europe, North America, the Near East and Australasia. In this country it grows mostly on waysides at the edges of cornfields and on scrubland.

The root of the plant is short, but it sends up stems of eight to 20 inches (20-50cm) long which are crowned with sprays of two—or three— feathered leaves. The flowerheads grow singly at the end of each divided stem and consist of a circle of white petals around a flower centre of four to five thousand yellow stamens.

**Harvesting tips:** The flowerhead is the

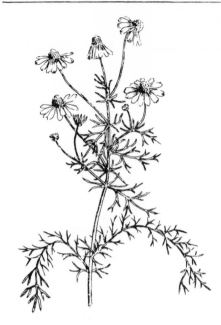

most important part of the plant for the home doctor, but its effectiveness depends a lot on the method of harvesting and drying. The best time for harvesting is between the third and fifth day after flowering, because then most of the medically useful substances in the flower are at their peak. Drying should preferably take place in controlled drying rooms as there should be plenty of air and the temperature should not be too high. For a camomile bath it is best to harvest the whole plant (again while it is in bloom) and hang it up in bundles to dry in an airy place.

**Active contents:** Recent research has established that camomile possesses certain properties that render poisonous bacteria harmless, which means that it can be administered in infectious illnesses caused, for example, by staphylococci or streptococci. This is a scientific fact which explains its good results against infections, and proves its usefulness as a steam inhalant for bronchial disorders.

The most important constituent of camomile is its essential oils, two of which—chamazulene and bisabolol—are agents against inflammation and especially effective in treating the stomach wall. Other healing agents in the essential oils of camomile are flavone-glycosides and coumarin which are useful for the relief of cramps.

Camomile can be taken internally for acute stomach pains because it will calm the stomach and quickly bring complete relief. For cases of chronic inflammation of the stomach wall and stomach ulcers, camomile tea is also to be recommended. One unsweetened cupful should be taken three times a day before meals. For complaints of the gall bladder add peppermint and balm to the tea. If the stomach upset is of nervous origin, balm and camomile are to be recommended in equal proportions.

**To prepare camomile tea:** Pour a cupful of hot water over one to two teaspoonsful of camomile flowers and let it draw for ten minutes before straining. The tea should be drunk warm but not too hot. If you have a cold, or inflammation of the nose and throat, then inhaling the steam from camomile tea can be most soothing.

Camomile can also be used externally on slow-healing wounds. Immerse the affected area into an infusion of camomile flowers, or soak a clean cloth in the infusion, gently binding the wound with it. Both methods are recognized as being equally effective and were used by military doctors at one time. However, in cases of bad open wounds it is essential to consult your doctor who may advise an injection against tetanus.

**To prepare a steam bath of camomile:** Put a handful of flowers into a bowl and pour over them two pints (1 litre) of boiling water. Bend over the bowl and cover both the bowl and your head with a large towel to keep the steam in. Inhale for five to ten minutes.

**An important warning:** Camomile is one of those healing plants which must not be taken in overdose because it may cause nervous disturbance, dizziness or even conjunctivitis. It should therefore not be taken in large doses over a long period of time.

## CARAWAY

*Carum carvi*     Family: Umbelliferae

**Part used:** Dried fruit (*Fructus carvi*).
**Helps:** Flatulence, stomach ache.
**Description:** Although caraway grows wild all over Europe and in the Near East, it is mostly cultivated for use in the kitchen and the medicine cabinet. This no doubt ensures a higher quality of plant and a finer aroma. Caraway has a spindle-shaped root and an upright and many-branched stalk that grows up to a yard (1 metre) high. The stalks are forked, and the leaves feathered and sometimes red in colour. The umbels have from seven to ten ribs.

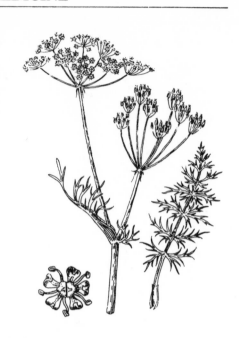

**Active contents:** Caraway's essential oils are its most important healing agents and these consist of limonene, carveol, dihydrocarvone and up to 60 per cent carvone. Caraway is the best of all the healing plants to use in the treatment of flatulence. For more details of its use see under Aniseed.

## CENTAURY

*Erythraea*     Family:
*centaurium*     Gentianaceae

**Part used:** Whole plant (*Herba centaurii*).
**Helps:** Loss of appetite and indigestion due to lack of digestive juices. Also regulates the gall bladder.
**Description:** This is a delicate and not immediately obvious plant found in woodland clearings and on damp mea-

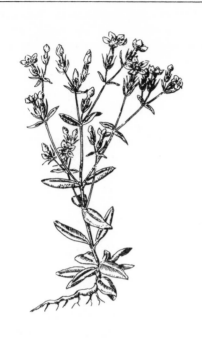

dowland. It has a tap-root and a four-cornered stem that can grow from four to twenty inches (10-50cm) tall. The stalk springs from a rosette of leaves often not visible because it grows at ground level and is usually hidden by grass. The leaves on the stem alternate, and the flowers arranged in forked panicles. The five-petalled calyx supports the white tulip-shaped base of the flower which ends in five pointed red petals that only open to form a star-shaped bloom when the sun is shining. Centaury belongs to the gentian family and is acidic by nature.

**Harvesting tips:** The whole plant is used and should be harvested while it is in bloom. Hang it up in bundles in an airy place to dry. It will be noticed that the stem is the most bitter part of the plant, and the leaves the least bitter.

**Active contents:** Glycosidic bitter matter is responsible for the pharmacological effects of this plant. Centaury is a very bitter plant the medical applications of which are similar to that of Gentian (see page 55).

**To prepare centaury tea:** This tea works best when made with cold water. Take a heaped teaspoonful of centaury to every cup and leave to stand in the cold water for six to ten minutes. Drink a cupful at room temperature before each meal. It has been found to be especially beneficial in cases of *anorexia nervosa.*

Although there are more effective plants for treating acute complaints of the stomach and intestines, centaury is to be highly recommended for chronic gastritis and countless disorders (like loss of appetite and indigestion) which stem from the lack of gastric juices. All these conditions result ultimately from nervous exhaustion. The effect of the centaury spreads to the intestines and will even be felt in the gall bladder.

## COLTSFOOT

*Tussilago farfara*                    Family: Compositae

**Part used:** Leaves (*Folia farfarae*)
**Helps:** Irritating coughs and chronic bronchitis. Especially good if the patient has pneumoconiosis or emphysema.
**Description:** Coltsfoot is to be found all over Europe and Northern and Central Asia. In this country it prefers moist loamy soil. The yellow fingers begin to bloom as early as February, although they only open when the sun

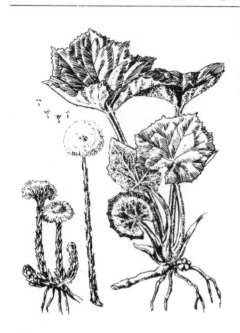

shines. The flowers are not as valuable to medicine as the leaves, which appear much later.

**Harvesting tips:** The best time to collect the leaves is during May, June and July, when they are as big as saucers. They should be chopped up before they are dried and stored.

**Active contents:** The main healing agent in coltsfoot is mucilage (see page 26). There is also some bitter matter and a small amount of tannin.

**To prepare coltsfoot tea:** Take two teaspoonsful of chopped coltsfoot leaves to each cupful of water, boil the mixture and strain after allowing it to stand for about ten minutes.

Although coltsfoot has been used for centuries as a remedy for coughs it is becoming more valued by modern medicine in the treatment of pneum-oconiosis and emphysema. Neither of these diseases can be cured, and so anything that affords relief is to be doubly welcomed. One of the worst features of both diseases is the terrible coughing attacks which start the day. These can be brought on by the slightest disturbance—even getting out of bed will cause them—so it is a good idea to prepare coltsfoot tea the night before and put in on the bedside table in a thermos flask. Plenty of honey in the tea also helps.

When it is not being used on its own for a special purpose, coltsfoot makes a good addition to almost any herbal tea.

Other plants which are similar to coltsfoot in both constituents and effect are ribwort plantain (*Plantago lanceolata*), Icelandic moss (*Cetraria islandica*), marshmallow (*Althaea officinalis*) and mallow (*Malva silvestris*). All these are likely to be found in herbal teas treating coughs. Butterbur (*Petasites hybridus*) was also widely used at one time for treating coughs, but now it is more readily recommended for nervous disorders of the stomach and gall bladder, especially when combined with wormwood (¾ oz/20g wormwood and 1 oz/30g butterbur leaves).

**An important warning:** It is always important when suffering from a cough to determine the actual cause of the complaint: the cough itself is merely a symptom. However, the cough has its uses and is the most efficient way of getting rid of phlegm. If the patient begins to cough blood, has a temperature or sweats heavily at

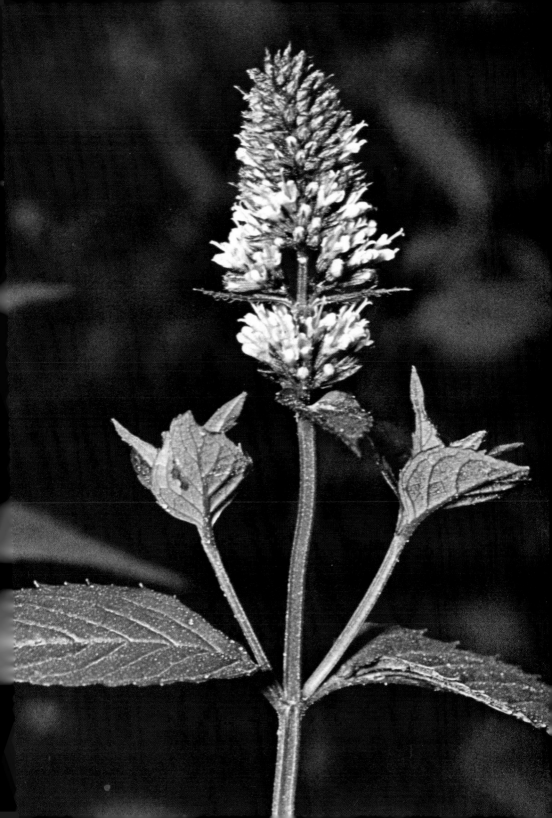

*Top left:* Butterbur  *Top right:* Tormentil
*Bottom left:* Lungwort  *Bottom right:* Comfrey

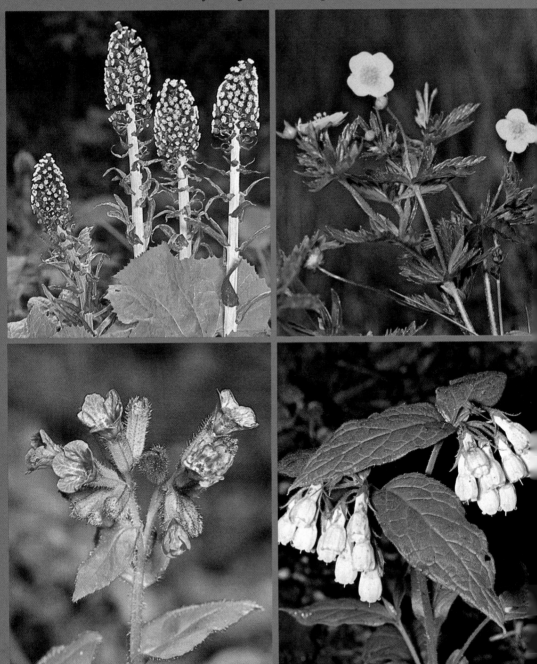

night, or if the cough lasts for more than two weeks, a doctor should always be consulted.

## COMFREY

*Symphytum officinale*

Family: Boraginaceae

**Part used:** Root (*Radix symphyti/ Radix consolidae*).

**Helps:** Heal ulcers, broken bones and weeping wounds.

**Description:** Comfrey is a member of the borage family and grows in profusion in damp and shady places such as on the banks of ditches and at the edge of woodland. Its stalks and leaves are covered with rough hairs and its bell-shaped flowers vary in colour from pink through violet to white.

**Active contents:** The main healing agent is allantoin, but comfrey root also contains tannin, starch and other matter. The allantoin increases the secretion of the wound so that the pus is able to flow away, and it also stimulates the blood to form a scab.

**To make a solution of comfrey:** Take 3½ oz (100g) comfrey root and boil it in 2 pints (1 litre) of water for ten minutes. Strain the liquid and use it in warm compresses.

## COWSLIP

*Primula veris*

Family: Primulaceae

**Part used:** Root (*Radix primulae*) and flowers (*Flos primulae*).

**Helps:** Coughs caused by phlegm.

**Description:** The cowslip is a perennial plant of the primrose family which can be found in meadowland. Its bright yellow bell-like flowers bloom in April and May.

**Active contents:** Healing plants which contain saponin are invaluable in the treatment of stubborn coughs hampered by phlegm, and the roots of cowslip are rich in it, as well as containing essential oils and glycosides. Cowslip flowers also contain some saponin.

The roots of the cowslip are a common ingredient in herbal teas and extracts of the root are often found in cough linctus. Cowslip is especially effective in treating chronic bronchitis and the severe racking coughs often suffered by the elderly.

An excellent tea for troublesome coughs can be made from three parts cowslip to two parts of aniseed, fennel and coltsfoot. Take two teaspoonsful

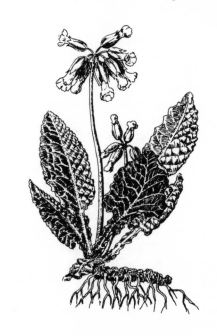

of the tea mixture and pour boiling water over it. Strain after allowing to stand for ten minutes, sweeten with honey and drink hot.

Other plants that are suitable for treating coughs are Great Mullein (*Verbascum thapsus*) and Lungwort (*Pulmonaria officinalis*). If the cough is spasmodic, Thyme (*Thymus vulgaris*) and Sundew (*Drosera rotundifolia*) are to be recommended. Thyme is best known as a culinary herb, but apart from its delightful smell and taste it contains essential oils which relieve cramps.

## DANDELION

*Taraxacum officinale*      Family: Compositae

**Part used:** Root and leaves (*Radix taraxaci cum herba*).

**Helps:** Chronic rheumatic and arthritic complaints, gall stones, kidney stones. Also stimulates the metabolism.

**Description:** The dandelion is an unfussy plant that will grow anywhere regardless of the soil type. Its strong tap-root, which descends down to a foot (30cm) into the ground, makes it very difficult to uproot as all gardeners with lawns will know. The dandelion has a rosette of leaves, lance-shaped and 2 to 10 inches (5-25cm) long with irregularly toothed edges. Its yellow flowers are round composite heads on longish hollow stalks.

**Harvesting tips:** Uproot the plant and cut the tap-root in half lengthwise. Hang root and leaves up to dry, then cut them up together.

The dandelion is a plant as beautiful as it is useful, and were it not for the fact that it is so troublesome on lawns and in cultivated gardens, it would no doubt take its place in the flower border alongside existing plants. Its leaves are delicious in salads and its 'clocks' a delight to children.

**Active contents:** The dandelion contains plenty of vitamins, especially vitamin C and B2, and a variety of minerals and trace elements which are all necessary for life. It also contains acids which are vital for digestion and act as a tonic on the stomach and other digestive organs. All these substances working together in the dandelion stimulate the metabolism in an effective way.

**To prepare dandelion tea:** Pour a cupful of water over one to two teaspoonsful chopped dandelion, bring to

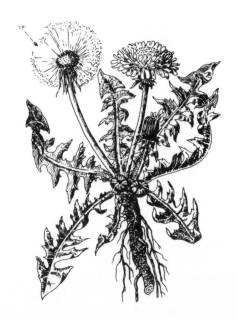

the boil and take it off the heat after one minute. Let the tea brew for ten minutes before straining. Drink a cupful in the morning and a cupful in the evening every day for four to eight weeks for a tonic that will be of particular help to those suffering from rheumatism and arthritis.

Dandelion is not only useful as a general tonic—it can also be used to treat specific illnesses, and recent research suggests that it can prevent the formation of gall stones. Since milk thistle is also excellent for the gall bladder, a very good tea can be made with equal amounts of this and dandelion.

The dandelion is also diuretic—that is it stimulates the flow of urine. It can be used, as well, in the treatment of kidney stones and as a prophylactic against new ones forming.

In the treatment of rheumatic conditions juniper berries can be used to augment the use of the dandelion, and it is suggested that one berry is taken three times a day, followed by twenty-five berries three times a day, then back to one berry on alternate days.

### DOG ROSE

*Rosa canina*  
Family: Rosaceae

**Part used:** Ripe fruit (*Fructus cynosbati*).  
**Helps:** Colds and fevers.  
**Description:** The wild rose, from which our garden roses have been developed, is to be found growing in hedgerows and along fences and roadsides. It is a bushy plant with flat pink flowers which have no smell and bloom in June and July. In late summer and early autumn the red rose hips are formed, and when these are cut open hard kernels (*semen cynosbati*) are visible inside. The red fleshy fruit (*fructus cynosbati*) can be used alone or together with the kernels, which contain a small amount of vanilla, and make the tea taste very pleasant.

**Harvesting tips:** It is very easy to collect rose hips in autumn from the hedgerows. You should only pick the thoroughly ripe fruit, which should be bright red. Cut up the fruit to dry them.

**Active contents:** The fleshy part of the rose hip is very rich in vitamin C, and it also contains other important vitamins from the B group, vitamin A, E and K, as well as trace elements, fructose, acids, tannin and pectin.

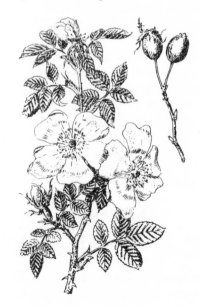

This richness makes it a very useful fruit and the tea made from it not only tastes good, it actually does good to those suffering from the common cold, and strengthens patients in the grip of fever. This is because vitamin C helps in building resistance to disease. Vitamin C cannot be retained in the body and when you have a temperature it is used up especially quickly, so it is essential to ensure that your diet contains sufficient of this important vitamin.

**To prepare rose hip tea:** For 1½ pints (¾ litre) of tea you will need ½ oz (15g) or two teaspoonsful finely chopped rose hip. Pour water over the hips, bring to the boil and cook for ten minutes.

Rose hips go well with almost all other healing plants and a little rose hip added to any other tea will improve both its taste and its medicinal value. To make a tea which will act as a gentle laxative and diuretic, take ¾ oz (20g) rose hips with kernels and mix with ¾ oz (20g) Alder Buckthorn bark to a cupful of water and either boil for five minutes or bring quickly to the boil and let the tea draw for twenty minutes.

Another useful remedy for infections, fever, general debility and the healing of wounds is blackcurrant (*ribes nigrum*). The cold juice should be diluted with hot water.

## EYEBRIGHT

*Euphrasia*  Family:
*officinalis*  Scrophulariaceae

**Part used:** Whole plant.
**Helps:** Acutely and chronically inflamed eyes, stinging and weeping eyes, over-sensitivity to light.

**Description:** Eyebright grows in mountainous and flat regions, but it is happiest on dry meadow and moorland or woodland clearings. The plant grows up to twelve inches (30cm) high and it blooms in late summer and autumn. Its delicate pale violet flowers, which spring singly from the leaf axes, are veined with dark violet and display a yellow speckle on the lower lip. The stalk is covered with downy hairs and the leaves, which grow in opposite pairs, are about half an inch (1cm) long and egg-shaped, ending in two or three teeth.

**Harvesting tips:** Gather the whole plant while it is in bloom in late summer or autumn, and dry in bundles in an airy place.

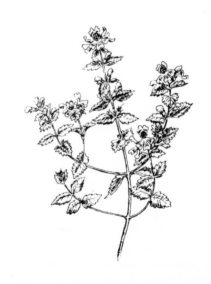

**To prepare eyebright tea:** Add a teaspoonful of the chopped plant to a cupful of water and bring to the boil. Leave to draw for two minutes before adding a couple of crystals of cooking salt. The salt will make the liquid more compatible with the salt water in the eyes.

Another useful tea can be made by mixing ¼ oz (10g) fennel with ½ oz (15g) camomile and 1 oz (25g) eyebright. Put a heaped teaspoonful in a cup and pour on boiling water. Leave to draw for fifteen minutes. This tea is equally good as a drink and for compresses.

Eyebright tea applied on a compress is very effective against the most varied of eye complaints, including conjunctivitis and blepharitis (inflammation of the edge of the eyelid). In fact, any injury to the eye is helped by its soothing effect. Sties can be treated with warm compresses of equal amounts of eyebright and camomile, and eyebright tea dropped directly into the eye will ease irritation of tired and burning eyes and minimize sensitivity to light. Taken internally the tea will strengthen immunity to these complaints.

Eyebright is one of the few plants whose usefulness has not been exaggerated by folklore. Delicate children who are especially prone to catching coughs and colds and often suffer from watering eyes at the slightest suspicion of a draught used to be called 'scrofulus children' because of their receptiveness to this plant. Indeed, their general health can be greatly improved if given an eyebath of eyebright tea first thing in the morning and last thing at night, with half a pint (¼ litre) of eyebright tea to drink during the day. If taken regularly this cure will prove most effective over a period of months.

## FENNEL

*Foeniculum vulgare*                Family: Umbelliferae

**Part used:** Dried fruit (*Fructus foeniculi*).

**Helps:** Wind, stomach cramps, coughing.

**Description:** Fennel can be either annual or perennial. It may die down in winter or it may survive to the next year. It grows from three to six feet (1-2 metres) tall on a long round stalk ribbed with blue, and it divides at the top to form feathery leaves with three or four fingers and composite umbels of tiny yellow flowers.

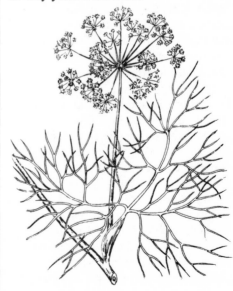

Fennel is cultivated over almost all of Europe and, although it originated in the Mediterranean, it is now quite at home in Britain and enjoys as much popularity in the kitchen as it does in the medicine chest. A variant of this is the vegetable fennel, a delicious accompaniment to fish which is now to be found in most good greengrocers and supermarkets.

**Active contents:** In both cookery and medicine only the seeds of fennel are used. They are rich in essential oils and very similar to aniseed in that they contain 50 to 60 per cent anethole. For the application of fennel see under Aniseed (page 39).

### FIELD HORSETAIL

*Equisetum*　　　　　　Family:
*arvense*　　　　　　Equisetaceae

**Part used:** Young stems (*Herba equiseti*).

**Helps:** Rheumatism and general circulation trouble and can be administered externally in the form of a silicic acid bath or taken internally, especially for chilblains or swellings resulting from broken bones.

**Description:** Field horsetail is found in spring in woodland clearings and ditches where it grows in damp loamy soil. It is also plentiful on wasteland and at the edges of cultivated fields. It grows from a thin rhizome, and in spring sends up vertical brownish shoots which carry the ears or seed heads. A few weeks later these are followed by the green growth; a stalk which can reach eight to twelve inches (20-30cm) in height and is ringed by

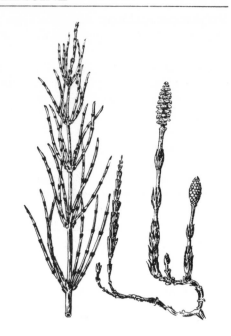

rosettes of green sideshoots. It is the green growth which is used in plant medicine.

**Harvesting tips:** The best time to collect horsetail is in early summer. Cut the plant just above the ground and hang it in bundles to dry in an airy place. In recent years the plant has been recommended for its slightly diuretic properties and is prescribed for rheumatism and gout, as a compress for slow-healing wounds, as a mouthwash and as an addition to bath water.

**Active contents:** The field horsetail contains silicic acid, flavonoids and saponins. These last two work together to produce a slightly diuretic effect, and are the reason why the field horsetail is used in teas and infusions to treat the kidneys, though it is not a strong enough diuretic to be used on its own. However, the most important ingredient is the silicic acid, which aids the circulation. Taken in a tea, or applied externally in the form of a solution, it will have an immediate local effect which will build up gradually as the dose is repeated.

Field horsetail baths accelerate the metabolic rate through the skin and are therefore especially effective for circulation troubles, swellings caused by broken bones and chilblains. The pain caused by rheumatic diseases and gout is also relieved by this treatment.

**To prepare the bath:** Steep about 3½ oz (100g) of field horsetail in hot water for an hour to draw, and then add the liquid to the bath water. Extracts of the plant can sometimes be bought for this purpose and are to be strongly recommended.

Teas and infusions made from the field horsetail are effective against rheumatic diseases, chronic coughs and kidney trouble. Use it, too, as a blood-purifying agent.

**To prepare the tea:** Use one to two teaspoonsful of the cut plant to one cupful of water. If the water is cold allow to steep for twelve hours, but if the water is hot thirty minutes will be sufficient. Drink three cupsful per day and don't expect a miracle cure; the drug will take a long time to build up in your body.

## GENTIAN

*Gentiana*              Family:
*lutea*                 Gentianaceae

**Part used:** Root (*Radix gentianae*).
**Helps:** Loss of appetite and complaints

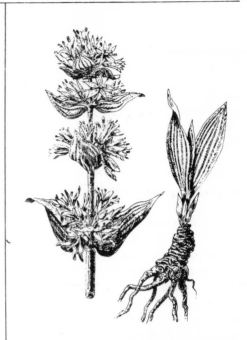

of the stomach and intestine caused by insufficient digestive juice.

**Description:** The tall yellow gentians the roots of which are used in medicine look very different from the blue flowers so often seen on postcards of the Alps. If you want to use the gentian in home medicine you will have to buy the cultivated root from druggists. Even if you are in the Alps you will not be able to dig it up as it is now very rare and a protected species.

**Active contents:** The gentian belongs to the group of plants that contain *amara tonica,* pure bitter drugs. Its other constiuents are of lesser importance and it contains very little tannin indeed, which makes it most suitable for the treatment of stomach complaints. Loss of appetite, a feeling of fullness caused by insufficient digestive juice, wind and cramps in the stomach and intestine can all be effectively treated with gentian tea or tincture of gentian. The acidic contents of the plant (gentiopicrine and the newly discovered amarogentine) activate healing influences as soon as they touch the mucous membrane inside the mouth, but they are also absorbed and continue to be effective internally.

**To prepare gentian tea:** Pour 1½ pints (¾ litre) water over a teaspoonful of gentian root and brew for five minutes. The tea should be drunk warm, but not hot, before meals and at any time when the patient is suffering from acute stomach pains resulting from a feeling of fullness. Gentian can also be mixed with Lesser Centaury in equal proportions and it can be bought like this in the shops.

Before taking the dose it is important to identify the exact nature of the stomach complaint. If the digestive juices are not plentiful enough then gentian is the answer, but if the stomach is over-acidic, then it should be avoided. In these cases you should resort to Balm, Caraway, Camomile and Aniseed, which can also be mixed with a light sedative like Valerian or St John's Wort.

### GREATER CELANDINE

*Chelidonium*          Family:
*majus*            Papaveraceae

**Part used:** Whole plant (*Herba chelidonii*).
**Helps:** Complaints of the gall bladder, stomach cramps, swollen liver. The

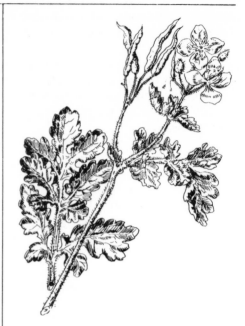

yellow milky sap from the fresh celandine can remove warts.
**Description:** The greater celandine is always found near human habitation, on roadsides, hedgerows, old walls and cultivated land. It blooms throughout the warmer months of the year and its lively yellow flowers, the yellow milky sap in its stem and its bluish green leaves make it unmistakable. Its seed pods hold oily seeds very much sought after by ants, and for this reason the greater celandine is to be found growing in the most unusual places such as steep walls or the turrets of old castles. The plant belongs to the poppy family.
**Harvesting tips:** The best time to collect this plant is in the early autumn, as long as it is still in flower. Dry the herb as quickly as possible in an airy place.

This plant has long been known for its healing properties, and records from before the time of Christ show that, even then, it was used to treat jaundice, swelling of the liver, gallstones and constipation. It has treated the same complaints ever since in folk medicine and, although rejected for a long time by orthodox medicine, we know enough about it today to be able to use it to its best advantage to treat the same complaints.

**Active contents:** Greater celandine contains essential oils and its yellow milky sap contains the antibacteriae alkaloids chelidonine, chelerythrine, sanguinarine and berberine, amongst others. These contents indicate that celandine acts as a gentle sedative and relieves cramp in the bronchial tubes, the intestine and the gall bladder. It also raises the blood pressure slightly. These properties make celandine ideal in any teas designed for the treatment of the gall bladder or liver.

**To prepare greater celandine tea:** Take two teaspoonsful of celandine to a cupful of hot water. Let the tea draw for ten minutes and drink it warm.

One of the reasons why the celandine has not always been trusted by medical science, in spite of its remarkable properties, is that the quantity of active drugs in the plant varies from season to season. Plants harvested in the spring, or those which have been stored for longer than six months often have only a tenth of the potency they should have.

Another remarkable property of celandine is the way its yellow milky sap can be used to remove warts. They do in fact disappear when dabbed repeatedly with this sap and in some cases very quickly indeed. However, this is not a reliable treatment and why it works on some people but not on others has yet to be discovered.

## HAWTHORN

*Craetaegus oxycantha*  Family: Rosaceae

**Part used:** Flowers (*Flos crataegi*).
**Helps:** Palpitations and heart strain due to old age.
**Description:** The hawthorn blooms in May and June. It is a member of the rose family and its white flowers are arranged in panicles. As the name suggests, the branches of the hawthorn tree are covered in sharp thorns. The

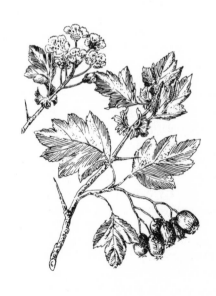

leaves are mostly three-lobed with irregular saw edges, dark green on the upper side and light to bluish green on the underside. They grow on short stalks close to the twig. Hawthorn can be found growing in almost any situation, but it is particularly fond of woods and hedges. The pink hawthorn, which is planted as an ornamental tree in gardens and parks is related to its white namesake and is said to have the same beneficial effect on the heart.

**Harvesting tip:** Collect the flowers while they are in full bloom, but don't worry if a stray leaf or two finds its way into your harvest—they are not harmful. Quick drying is to be recommended. Store the dried flowers in airtight jars and, as their potency tends to deteriorate, collect a fresh batch every year and discard the old stock.

**Active contents:** The most important constituents include flavonoids, choline, acetylcholine, aethalymine and triterpenic acids. However, these agents are of little individual importance in hawthorn's effect on the heart: their significance lies in their combination and their interaction upon one another.

**To prepare hawthorn tea:** Using two teaspoonsful of hawthorn blossoms to each cupful of water, heat up and allow to stand for twenty minutes. Strain and sweeten with honey if desired.

Hawthorn stimulates the heart, but it plays a very different role from that of Foxglove and Lily of the Valley, and this is why it can be recommended (but only under a doctor's supervision) for home treatment. As its effect on heart and circulation is very gradual it is both necessary and safe to take it over a long period of time.

At the first sign of heart trouble, however, the patient *must* go to the doctor and remain under his supervision until such time as he is pronounced healthy again. To try and treat oneself for a heart complaint without advice is senseless and irresponsible, and the same applies to patients with high blood pressure.

## HEARTSEASE

*Viola*                                    Family:
*tricolor*                              Violaceae

**Part used:** Whole plant (*Herba violae tricoloris*).

**Helps:** Skin complaints, milk crust, eczema.

**Description:** Heartsease is a member of the pansy family and is to be found growing wild in fields and meadows, as well as being a common garden weed. There are two types: *arvensis,* which has small yellowish-white flowers, and *vulgaris,* whose flowers are predominantly violet. Both kinds are useful to the home doctor.

**Harvesting tips:** Collect the plants while they are in bloom and hang them in bundles in an airy place to dry.

**Active contents:** It is difficult to do justice to this plant as its healing powers have not yet been fully investigated. However, it is certain that it can clear various skin diseases including milk crust and eczema in children and that it is also useful in treating dry coughs. It has been found to contain saponins, flavones (includ-

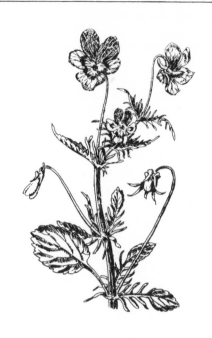

mixed together to make a tea to ward off colds and chills. Take a teaspoonful of the mixture per cup and pour over boiling water. Leave to draw for ten minutes and sweeten with honey if preferred.

## LIME

*Tilia*
*europoea*

Family:
Tiliaceae

**Part used:** Flowers (*Flos tiliae*).
**Helps:** Chills and influenza, where it is used to make the patient sweat and thus increase his natural resistance.
**Description:** The lime tree is so well known that it hardly needs describing, but few people know that there are two sorts of lime tree—the winter lime and the summer lime. The winter lime has

ing rutin), some salicylic acid compounds and calcium and magnesium salts.

**To prepare heartsease tea:** Pour a large cupful of hot water over two teaspoonsful of heartsease and allow to draw for ten minutes. Take three times a day.

When preparing food for babies and small children suffering from eczema or related skin problems it is a good idea to use heartsease tea instead of water. Older children and adults should take the tea for about four weeks after which there should be a noticeable improvement in even the most stubborn case of acne. Supplement the treatment with compresses and face packs made out of the tea.

Heartsease can also be taken in equal parts with Lime Blossom and

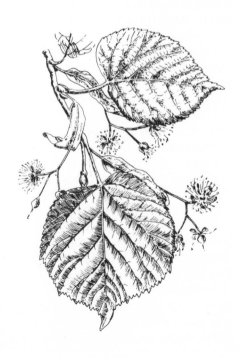

smaller leaves and more abundant blossoms than its summer counterpart. It is so named because it blooms about two weeks later than the summer lime. It is also more common. Another distinguishing factor is that on the underside of the leaves little tufts of hair grow in the axes of the veins. The hairs on the winter lime are yellowish-red, and those on the summer lime are white.

**Harvesting tips:** The medically useful part of the plant is the blossom, which can be collected from either type of lime tree. Collect the whole spray of flowers including the characteristic parchment-like leaf that grows from the flower stem, but make sure you do so within the first four days of blooming because this is when the flowers are at their most potent. Dry the flowers in an airy place at a temperature of not more than 113°F/45°C. Lime flowers are delicate things and after they have been dried and chopped they should be stored in tightly fitting jars that are light proof. Even the slightest damp will ruin the aroma of these flowers and will in turn lessen their potency.

**Active contents:** The pleasant smell of the lime flowers comes from the small amount of essential oils they contain, but their medical usefulness is due to flavonoid glycosides.

**To prepare lime blossom tea:** To induce sweating the tea needs to be a little stronger than normal. Pour half a pint (¼ litre) boiling water over two teaspoonsful of lime blossoms and strain after allowing to stand for ten minutes. Drink the tea very hot. For a preventative or enjoyable drink, take just one teaspoonful of flowers to a cup.

The fact that lime blossom induces sweating has been known for a very long time, it being especially used in the treatment of chills. Sweating increases the body's natural resistance to disease.

Lime blossom tea is also an excellent prophylactic. If you come home on a winter's evening frozen to the marrow, or have to walk a long way in the cold with wet feet, you will be likely to go down with a cold or feverish chill. But, if on arriving home you drink a cup of hot lime blossom tea, and a second three to four hours later, you will stand a good chance of waking up the next morning none the worse for wear.

Because of the tea's prophylactic qualities it is advisable to build up your resistance to colds by drinking it regularly when there is a lot of infection about. It tastes excellent and smells most pleasant and can be further enriched with honey if you prefer a sweeter drink.

Other remedies for chills include Elder flowers (*Flos sambuci*) from the Elder bush (*Sambucus nigra*). This is quite common in woods and on river banks, and its blossoms mixed in equal parts with lime blossom produces an excellent tea for sweating. As an extra tonic, Camomile and Wormwood can be added to these two ingredients. Each of the four plants should be taken in equal parts and mixed together. Take a heaped teaspoonful per cup and let the tea brew for about ten minutes before straining. Drink a cupful two or three times a day.

## LINSEED

*Linum*          Family:
*usitatissimum*          Linaceae

**Part used:** Seeds (*Semen lini*).

**Helps:** Constipation, inflammation of the mouth and throat, ulcers.

**Description:** Linseed, or flax, grows on a delicate stalk which bears alternate narrow lance-shaped leaves. In June and July sky-blue five-petalled flowers develop at the tips of the stalks and in the autumn the seed pods yield the flat, shiny, brown oval seeds.

**Active contents:** Linseed is a mild but effective laxative due to the oil and the glycoside linamarin that it contains. Its oily content makes it useful against inflammation, and it can be used as a gargle to relieve a sore throat, an irritating cough, or inflammation of the mouth. It can also be used as a poultice and applied to painful ulcers and boils.

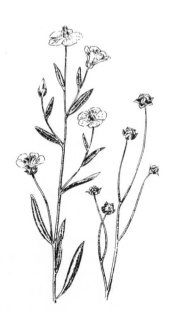

As a laxative, linseed should be taken crushed or ground. Do not soak the seeds first as they should swell only when they reach the intestine. If the seeds are mixed with fruit *purée* or sweetened with honey they are even more effective. Take two dessert-spoonsful of the mixture in the morning and in the evening. In general the bowels don't move immediately, and in severe cases of constipation two or three days can elapse before anything happens. Patience is needed as with all home remedies.

Medicinal linseed oil itself is a valuable addition to the home medicine chest and does much to ease the discomfort of many skin diseases like psoriasis and eczema, and relieves the extreme pain of shingles. Applied externally twice a day it will also help hasten the disappearance of warts and corns.

**To prepare linseed tea:** Pour a cupful of cold water over a teaspoonful of whole linseeds and allow to stand, stirring occasionally, for twenty minutes. Pour off the liquid and use it as a gargle or mouthwash, or as a tea, when it should be drunk lukewarm.

## MILK THISTLE

*Silybum*          Family:
*marianum*          Compositae

**Part used:** Fruit (*Fructus cardui mariae*).

**Helps:** Complaints of the liver.

**Description:** The milk thistle origin-

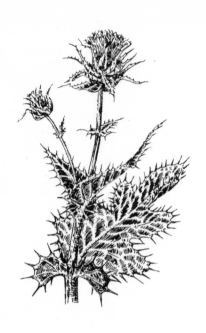

There is no doubt about the worth of milk thistle tea treatment for those with a tendency to liver trouble. Indeed, the tea is so effective that it has been known to minimize the after-effects of acute hepatitis (inflammation of the liver).

One rule that should not be broken, though, is that at the first sign of liver trouble you should consult your doctor. Symptoms include the whites of the eyes or the skin turning yellowish, faeces becoming white and urine brown.

**To prepare milk thistle tea:** Take a teaspoonful of milk thistle fruit and pour boiling water over it. Let it brew for ten to twenty minutes and strain. Slowly sip a cup of the hot tea three times a day: first thing in the morning; half an hour before lunch; and last thing at night. Do this for several weeks.

The tea can be mixed with Peppermint to improve its flavour and increase its effect.

## OAK

*Quercus robur*                    Family: Fagaceae

**Part used:** Bark (*Cortex quercus*).
**Helps:** Itching eyes; weeping eczema; leg ulcers.
**Active contents:** Oak bark contains tannin and has a strong astringent quality.
**To make oak bark tea:** Pour half a pint (¼ litre) of water over one to teaspoonsful of oak bark and boil for five minutes. Strain and use the liquid lukewarm. When applying on a compress over eczema and leg ulcers it is

ated in the Mediterranean region, but it has long been cultivated as a garden plant in Europe and the U.K. and it also grows wild here now. It has reddish-purple flowers and green and white marled leaves and makes a spectacular ornamental plant in any garden. The gleaming black or dark brown fruits with their hard husks are the medically useful part of the plant.
**Active contents:** The milk thistle contains flavonol silymarin, a drug which encourages the regeneration of liver cells and which can be taken in large doses without any fear of side-effects. It has been used in many experiments on animals and always with excellent results as it neutralizes the poisonous elements in many substances harmful to the liver.

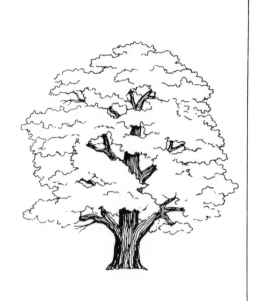

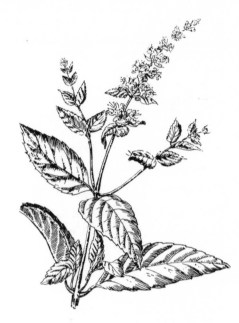

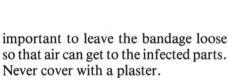

important to leave the bandage loose so that air can get to the infected parts. Never cover with a plaster.

## PEPPERMINT

*Mentha piperita*  Family: Labiatae

**Part used:** Leaves (*Folia menthae piperitae*).

**Helps:** Disorders of the stomach and intestines which give rise to vomiting and cramp; disorders of the gall bladder.

**Description:** Such a popular plant really needs no description. Its smell and taste are widely known, and of all the herbs used in cooking it is perhaps the one that most people know of. It can be found growing wild, but generally this plant is cultivated in the garden. It grows especially well in peat, but also thrives in a mixture of chalk and clay. Wild peppermint tends not to taste or smell as good as the cultivated kind, so it is best to grow your own. Every two years you should renew your stock of mint plants to ensure that the quality does not deteriorate.

**Active contents:** The main healing agent in peppermint is its essential oil which contains up to 60 per cent menthol. This acts as a light anaesthetic to the stomach wall, thereby taking away feelings of nausa and the desire to vomit. The acid in the plant also stimulates the gall bladder in conjunction with the essential oils, and its tannin content will soothe the inflammation in an irritated intestine.

**To prepare peppermint tea:** Pour a cupful of boiling water over a heaped teaspoonful of peppermint leaves, cover and let it draw for ten minutes. After straining it is best to drink the tea unsweetened as sugar interferes with the formation of acids.

Babies and very young children are often allergic to menthol so it is best to avoid giving them peppermint tea.

### ST JOHN'S WORT

*Hypericum*      Family:
*perforatum*      Hypericacae

**Part used:** Whole plant (*Herba hyperici*).

**Helps:** Depression and mild pains in the stomach, intestines and gall bladder. Also useful for healing wounds.

**Description:** St John's Wort has an unusual angular stalk and its leaves have a perforated appearance (hence *perforatum*). These 'perforations' are pores containing essential oil and resin. The flowers are yellow and five-petalled with many stamens.

**Harvesting tips:** Grows on sunny hillsides and slopes, on dry pastureland and at the edges of woods and roads. If you squash the yellow flowers it will stain your fingers bright red. This red dye can be seen as small dark points on the ends of the hairs inside the calyx and on the petals. Collect the upper part of the plant entire while it is blooming, around the end of June. Tie your harvest in bundles and hang up in airy place to dry.

**Active contents:** St John's Wort contains tannin, resin and essential oil. Its most important constituent, however, is hypericin, also called hypericum red. All these substances together activate the ducts of the digestive organs (and the gall bladder) and stimulate the circulation. Hypericin also acts as a gentle tranquillizer which helps cases of depression.

**To prepare oil of St John's wort:** You will need a plant which has just bloomed. Take about 4½ oz (125g) for every pint (½ litre) of water. Crush the flowers (a pestle and mortar is ideal for this), then add 18 fl oz (500ml) olive oil. Mix well and pour into a large clear glass jar with a wide neck. Leave the jar uncovered in a warm place and stir from time to time until fermentation

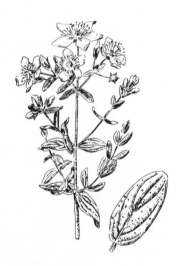

*Top left:* Coltsfoot    *Top right:* Haresfoot Clover
*Bottom left:* Sage    *Bottom right:* St John's Wort

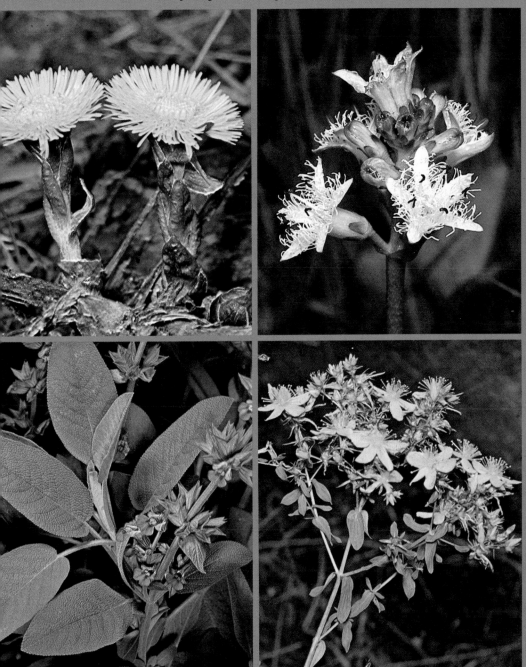

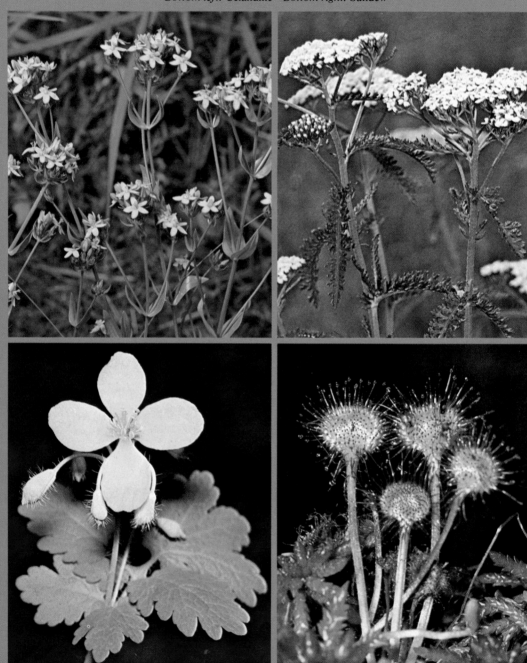

takes place. This will take about three to five days. Now put an airtight lid on the jar and keep it away from sunlight until the contents have taken on a luminous red colour (about six weeks). Pour off the oil, leaving the watery layer beneath, into airtight bottles. You can now use the oil both internally and externally.

Applied externally and rubbed into the skin it can relieve the pain of rheumatism and lumbago, as well as help heal wounds and dull pain. Soak a fine cotton handkerchief in oil of St John's wort and bind it around sprains, strained muscles and slow-healing wounds.

Taken internally, oil of St John's wort stimulates the gall bladder and calms a nervously upset stomach. Take a teaspoonful two to three times a day and continue the treatment over a long period if necessary. When treating depression with the oil you will also need to prolong the treatment as the real benefits only start to make themselves felt after two to three weeks.

**To prepare St John's wort tea:** Pour a cupful of water over two teaspoonsful of dried and chopped plant and bring to the boil. Strain after a few minutes. The tea should be taken twice or three times a day over a period of several weeks. There is no danger of harmful side-effects, but it is advisable to avoid contact with strong sunlight as St John's wort makes you extra sensitive to light.

Treatment with the tea is preferable to treatment with the oil because the tea retains a greater proportion of the healing agents.

## SWEET FLAG

*Acorus calamus*

Family: Araceae

**Part used:** Rhizome (*Radix calami*).

**Helps:** Nervous stomach upsets; mild liver and gall bladder complaints; loss of appetite. In a bath it can help nervous exhaustion.

**Description:** The sweet flag grows wild near slow running or stagnant water and in the mud it develops a long, fleshy creeping rhizome. From this grow leaves of up to 3 feet (1 metre) long which rise above the surface of the water. In June or July the plant

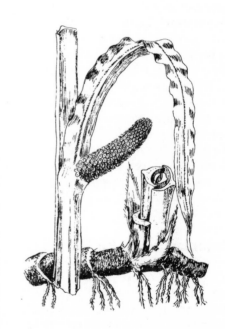

flowers, but the climate prevents the formation of fruit, and the plant, instead, reproduces through its rhizome.

**Harvesting tips:** Harvest the root of the plant in June or July. After it has been thoroughly cleaned, peel and cut in half, then lay out to dry. When completely dried out, chop the rhizome and store it in airtight jars away from direct sunlight.

**Active contents:** The most important healing agents in sweet flag are its essential oils and bitter matter. It belongs to the aromatic bitter tasting group of plants (*amara aromatica*)— see page 24). Its tannin content is too small to cause any irritation and acts only as a catalyst. Sweet flag is ideal for the treatment of the stomach, intestine and gall bladder and in cases of loss of appetite where general stimulation of the digestive processes is necessary.

When stomach upsets are of a nervous origin, or can be explained in psychological terms, sweet flag is a particularly suitable remedy.

**To prepare sweet flag tea:** Boil up half a pint (¼ litre) of water with two teaspoonsful of chopped and peeled sweet flag root and let the brew draw for fifteen minutes. Strain and drink lukewarm.

**To prepare a sweet flag bath:** To make your own extract of sweet flag, take 4 oz (100g) of unpeeled root, boil it for ten minutes in two pints (1 litre) of water and then strain. The liquid left will be enough for a full bath. This will act as a mild stimulant and it is a good antidote for exhaustion and aids convalescence after illness.

# TORMENTIL

*Potentilla erecta*        Family: Rosaceae

**Part used:** Root (*Radix tormentillae*).

**Helps:** Acute and chronic diarrhoea, and can be used as a gargle or mouthwash against inflammation of the mouth and throat.

**Description:** Tormentil belongs to the rose family and grows equally well in dry sandy soil or moist peat. The rhizome is the medically useful part of the plant, and from this grow a few three-to five-fingered leaves at the base of the flower stalks, which are leaved and topped with small yellow flowers.

**Harvesting tips:** An easy way to recognize tormentil is to count its petals: there are only four. When the rhizome is cut through it will quickly turn red.

**Active contents:** This plant is one of the richest in tannin (see page 25) of all native plants. It contains about 20 per cent catechol tannin (does not irritate the stomach). The tannin determines the red colour of the cut root and is probably responsible for minimizing bacteria and increasing the effectiveness of the plant.

There are two methods of taking tormentil: externally as a gargle or mouthwash against inflammation of the mouth, gums and tonsils, or internally for acute and chronic diarrhoea and flatulence caused by stomach upsets.

**To prepare tormentil tea:** Pour a pint (½ litre) water over one to three dessertspoonsful chopped tormentil rhizome and boil for fifteen minutes.

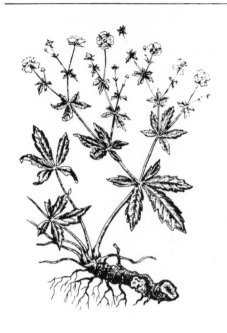

## VALERIAN

*Valeriana*  Family:
*officinalis*  Valerianaceae

**Part used:** Rhizome (*Radix valerianae*).

**Helps:** Nervous complaints, including palpitations; insomnia.

**Description:** Valerian grows in damp meadowland and woodland and on river banks. It can reach three feet (1 metre) in height and bears opposite pairs of feathered leaves and composite umbelliferous flowers with tiny pale or dark pink petals.

**Harvesting tips:** The root of this plant is its medicinally valuable part, and this should be dug up in September. Wash the root thoroughly and remove the fibrous root-hairs. An old comb is ideal for this job. Hang up the main

Drink three cupsful a day as required. The infusion can also be used as a gargle.

Another useful herb in the treatment of inflamed mouths, throats and tonsils is Sage, which contains antiseptic essential oils as well as tannin. Pour a cupful of boiling water over a heaped teaspoonful of sage leaves and strain after fifteen minutes. Gargle with this liquid three to five times a day.

Sage (*Salvia officinalis*) is a very old healing plant which originated in the Mediterranean region and has since become common in more northerly climes where it is often used for its flavour in cooking. Taken in concentrated doses (double the amount suggested above) it can control profuse sweating.

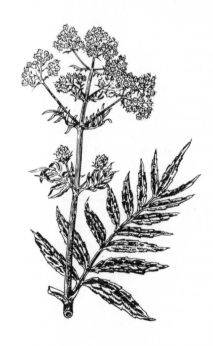

root to dry. As it dries it will give off the pleasant smell characteristic of valerian.

**Active contents:** Valerian contains an essential oil and alkaloids which combine to produce a calming sedative effect. Consequently valerian is useful in dealing with nervous complaints, and although it is prescribed as a tranquillizer it leaves the patient feeling refreshed rather than dopey.

Valerian can be taken in the form of a tea, a tincture, or as tablets containing an extract of valerian root. The tea is always more effective when made with cold water: on one hand less tannin will be absorbed and on the other the important healing agent is very sensitive to heat and can be completely destroyed by boiling.

**To prepare valerian tea:** Pour 1½ pints (1¼ litre) of cold water over two teaspoonsful of chopped valerian root and leave it to stand for ten to twelve hours, stirring from time to time. Drink the tea tepid two or three times a day.

A good tranquillizer can be made from equal quantities of valerian root and balm leaves. To prepare the tea, heat it up and then let it stand covered for about an hour. Use the same recipe, substituting hops for balm, for an effective sleeping draught.

**To prepare a valerian bath:** Take 4 oz (100g) valerian root and let it soak in two pints (1 litre) of water for ten hours. Remove the root and add the liquid to your bath water.

Another good treatment for nervous upsets is a lavendar bath. This can be taken alone or with rosemary and balm, and its delightful perfume has an effect that is both calming and stimulating. The nerves sensitive to smell transmit their reaction to the brain and so the beneficial effects are felt from within as well as externally.

To make your own lavendar, rosemary and balm bath, take about 2 oz (50g) of the plant material, which can be mixed to suit your own liking, add it to two pints (1 litre) of water, bring quickly to the boil and leave to stand for thirty minutes before straining and adding to your bathwater.

Lavendar tea is a light sedative which is particularly beneficial to the gall bladder, and rosemary acts as a tonic to the circulation and strengthens the heart.

## WORMWOOD

*Artemisia*                          Family:
*absinthium*                      Compositae

**Part used:** Whole plant (*Herba absinthii*).

**Helps:** Disorders of the stomach, gall bladder and intestines; stimulates the production of the digestive juices; encourages the appetite and prevents flatulence.

**Description:** Wormwood is a hardy plant that grows on stoney uncultivated land like scree and cliffs. Sideshoots branch from the main upright stem which is woody at the bottom and grows to a height of three feet (1 metre), and both stems and leaves are covered with fine silver-grey hairs. The leaves are feathery and three-fingered and the tiny round yellow flowers are arranged in forked panicles.

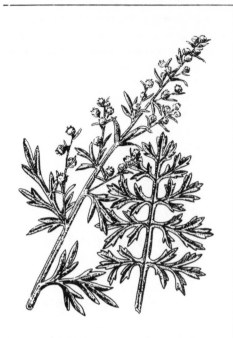

stand for ten minutes. Strain and drink a cupful three times a day after meals, making sure that it is good and warm (or drink a cupful whenever necessary). Don't be put off by its bitter taste, and don't try sweetening it as this robs it of some of its effectiveness. If, though, you find you cannot bear the bitter taste, mix it with Lesser Centaury and Peppermint in equal quantities. Take a teaspoonful of this mixture to a cupful of hot water and, after allowing to stand for five minutes, strain and use.

Other plants that help in a similar way to wormwood are Angelica (*Archangelica officinalis*) and St Benedict's Herb (*Cnicus benedictus*).

## YARROW

| *Achillea* | Family: |
|---|---|
| *millefolium* | Compositae |

**Part used:** Whole plant (*Herba millefolii*).

**Helps:** Disorders of the stomach and intestines.

**Description:** Yarrow is a hardy plant that grows from eight to eighteen inches (20-45cm) high and is very common on dry meadowland and around the edges of cultivated fields. The flower stalk springs from a rosette of leaves and ends in flat umbels of white flowers which can sometimes be tinged with red.

**Harvesting tips:** Gather the whole plant when the flowers are in bloom (June to September) and hang it up in bundles in an airy place to dry. When dry, chop it up, discarding the thick parts of the stalk.

**Harvesting tips:** The flowers and young shoots of wormwood are its medicinally valuable parts, and these should be collected at the beginning of the flowering season. Hang the plant in bundles in an airy place to dry. Closely related to wormwood is mugwort, but this plant has a lesser content of bitter matter.

**Active contents:** Wormwood contains the bitter principle absinthin, essential oils including thujone, and some tannin. It is successful in the treatment of stomach and gall bladder complaints. To a lesser degree, wormwood is also effective against colds and 'flu. It belongs to the *tonicum amarum* group (see page 24).

**To prepare wormwood tea:** Put a teaspoonful of chopped wormwood into a cupful of boiling water and leave to

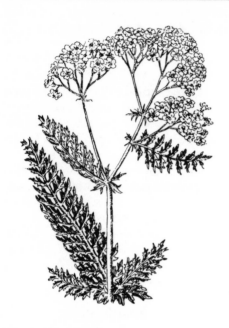

**Active contents:** Yarrow has many good qualities medicinally, and its combination of flavones, essential oils (including chamazulene) and tannins makes it useful in treating all sorts of stomach complaints (including loss of appetite since it encourages the gastric juices to flow) and disorders of the gall bladder and liver.

It is a very good remedy for 'tummy ache', but there are other plants which are more successful when it comes to dealing with gall bladder and liver troubles, and still others more efficient in dealing with stomach complaints like loss of appetite or flatulence: Wormwood; Gentian; Aniseed; Fennel; Caraway; Milk Thistle; Peppermint; Camomile and Greater Celandine, for instance. Unless you have a special preference for it, yarrow works best as an addition to other tea mixtures.

**To prepare yarrow tea:** Take a teaspoonful of chopped yarrow per cup and pour boiling water over it. Strain after leaving to stand for fifteen minutes and drink one cupful warm three times a day.

If you want a more potent yarrow tea, mix together one part of camomile, one part of peppermint and two parts of yarrow: you will find the results excellent.

**To prepare a yarrow bath:** Take 2-3 oz (50-75g) yarrow and pour over 2 pints (1 litre) of boiling water. Leave for twenty minutes, strain and add the liquid to your bath water.

# CHAPTER FIVE

# THE POTENT, THE EXOTIC AND THE NEW

In the previous section only those plants were described which it is possible to see on country walks. There were exceptions like arnica and gentian, which do not grow wild in this country, and others for which you may need a collector's licence, but on the whole the plants were all native ones.

This section deals with plants which are equally interesting to the home doctor but which, for one reason or another, you will need to buy ready-prepared from your health store or herbalist. If you want to try out any of these more unusual plants, it is essential to get the opinion of your doctor or herbalist first.

It features interesting facts about highly potent native plants; foreign plants which are increasingly being imported for use in home medicine, and garlic, ginseng, and devil's claw— three plants believed to have 'magic' powers.

## HIGHLY POTENT NATIVE PLANTS

### AUTUMN CROCUS

*Colchicum*       Family:
*autumnale*       Liliaceae

**Part used:** *Seeds (Semen colchici).*
This plant is to be found in late summer and autumn growing in moist meadowland and its pinky-lilac flowers are reminiscent of its springtime relative. It has wide lance-shaped leaves which grow up around the tall fruit-bearing stem. The seed pod is brown with three chambers which contain tiny blackish-brown seeds. Although the whole plant contains the alkaloid colchicine, only the seeds are used in the manufacture of drugs. Colchicine is a poison and overdoses can cause death. In pharmacy it is mainly used in the treatment of gout and can be successful when taken in measured doses.

## DEADLY NIGHTSHADE

*Atropa*                              Family:
*belladonna*                    Solanaceae

**Part used:** Leaves (*Folia belladonnae*).
Deadly nightshade is, as its name
would suggest, a deadly poisonous
plant which grows in woodland
clearings. All parts of the plant contain
the alkaloid atropine which, taken in
the right doses, can relieve cramp,
especially in the stomach and
intestines. Atropine is also used in eye
surgery: a few drops in the eye will
enlarge the pupil.

## ERGOT

*Claviceps*                           Family:
*purpurea*                    Hypocreaceae

**Part used:** Fungus (*Secale cornutum*).
Nowadays ergot is fortunately quite a
rare sight, but you may still be able to
spot it in a rye field: a dark violet
fungoid growth which feeds on the
grain. The seeds of this fungus contain
very potent alkaloids and if they are
not detected in time and end up being
milled with the grain they can cause
mass poisoning. There are gruesome
historical records of this happening.

It is still grown in laboratories by
major pharmaceutical companies
because its constituents have become
invaluable to medicine and in particular to gynaecology.

## FOXGLOVE

*Digitalis*                           Family:
*purpurea*              Scrophulariaceae

**Part used:** Leaves (*Folia digitalis*).
All types of foxglove contain substances invaluable to heart therapy.
The red and pink varieties grow wild in
English woodland, though the varieties used in pharmacology are grown
specially by the manufacturers.

## LILY OF THE VALLEY

*Convallaria*                         Family:
*majalis*                       Liliaceae

**Part used:** Whole plant (*Herba conval-
lariae*).
This sweet-smelling May flower is a
favourite for picking for the house.
Although it is poisonous, it can be very
beneficial to damaged heart muscles if
given in the right doses.

## POPPY

*Papaver*                             Family:
*somniferum*               Papaveraceae

**Part used:** Capsules (*Fructus papaveris
maturus*).
The opium poppy, a relative of the
garden poppy, does grow wild but is
mainly cultivated for medical use.
Opium is made from the milk sap of
the seed pod and the poppy is grown on
a very large scale in Asia Minor,
Macedonia and Persia for this
purpose. Opium contains very
valuable and important alkaloids, the
best known of which is morphine. It
was first isolated by a chemist called
Friedrich Sertürner in 1804. Since then

it has played a vital role as a painkiller, but it is also an addictive drug which today is prescribed only under the strictest supervision. Another derivative of opium is papaverine, which combats cramps in the digestive tract, and codeine, which has many medical uses, notably in the treatment of coughs.

## THORN APPLE

*Datura*  
*stramonium*

Family:  
Solanaceae

**Part used:** Leaves (*Folia stramonii*).  
Like deadly nightshade, the thorn apple thrives in darkness and is very poisonous. It gets its name from its prickly walnut-sized fruit. It is mostly cultivated for the drugs industry but can still be found growing wild, mainly on wasteland, and is recognizable by its large white funnel-shaped flowers. Its main healing agents are alkaloids, including hyoscyamine. The leaves and seeds are used to make a tincture that is often prescribed for asthma. The leaves are sometimes used in special cigarettes for asthmatics.

## FOREIGN PLANTS USED IN HOME MEDICINE

### ALOES

*Aloe*  
*vera*

Family:  
Liliaceae

Aloes is a purgative drug produced from the sap of the aloe tree. This is a bitter viscous juice found in the leaves which is dried out until all the fluid has been removed and a solid substance remains.

The aloe tree grows between 6½ to 10 feet (2 to 3 metres) high. At the top of its stem is a bush of lance-shaped, very fleshy leaves with dark purple thorns which can be up to two feet (60cm) long. The flower stalk is about three feet (1 metre) long and bears bunches of pale pink cylindrical flowers. Aloes contains anthrachinon and its derivatives aloin and resin, which are strong purgatives much used by the pharmaceutical industry. It is also used in medicines to treat the stomach and gall bladder.

### BALSAM OF TOLU

*Myroxylon*  
*balsamum*

Family:  
Leguminosae

**Part used:** Resin.  
Balsam tolu comes from a tree native to Central America that grows up to 52 feet (16 metres) high. The balsam is obtained in a most peculiar way. First the trunk of the tree is knocked hard near its base with a blunt instrument. Then the outer bark is peeled off and the wound 'sterilized' with flaming brands. After a few days the balsam begins to seep through and is collected by soaking it up in a cloth. After the first harvest a deeper cut is made into the bark and the same process repeated. The cloths are then heated along with various pieces of bark that have been removed from the tree, and the raw balsam produced then goes through various refining processes. The end product is a pleasant smelling, dark coloured and syrupy liquid that is used to heal all sorts of skin diseases. It can be found in various salves and

lotions and acts as a mild antiseptic; it is also a very effective treatment against itching haemorrhoids. Its pleasant smell is derived from its vanilla content, and it also contains cumarin and alkaloid resins.

## BITTER ORANGE

*Citrus*                    Family:
*aurantium*                 Rutaceae

**Part used:** Rind of fruit (*Pericarpium aurantii*).
The peel of the bitter orange from the Mediterranean is very different from the peel of an ordinary eating orange because it contains a very bitter aromatic essential oil. The bitter orange belongs to the *amara aromatica* group and tinctures made from its peel are added to many tonics and medicines which stimulate the digestion. Because of its pleasant smell even children can be persuaded to take it despite its bitterness.

## BOLDO

*Peumus*                    Family:
*boldus*                    Monimiaceae

**Part used:** Leaves (*Folia boldo*).
Boldo leaves are imported from Chile and have recently been incorporated into tea mixtures used to treat the stomach, intestines and gall bladder. They are rich in essential oils and boldine, an alkaloid which is an excellent stimulant to the digestive tract.

## CINCHONA

*Cinchona*                  Family:
*officinalis*               Rubiaceae

**Part used:** Bark (*Cortex chinae*).
The bark of the China tree contains quinine, which is well known for its successful treatment of malaria. Quinine is now available in pure form as a solid and is used in drugs prescribed to build up the strength and stimulate the appetite. The China tree is cultivated for the drugs industry in Java and Africa.

## CONDURANGO

*Marsdenia*                 Family:
*condurango*                Asclepiadaceae

**Part used:** Bark (*Cortex condurango*).
The condurango grows on the western slopes of the Cordillera in Ecuador. Its bark has a bitter taste and is used in medicine as an *amarum*. Today the drug itself is seldom used but condurango wine and other similarly bitter preparations are still used to stimulate the appetite and the digestion.

## EUCALYPTUS

*Eucalyptus*                Family:
*globulus*                  Myrtaceae

**Part used:** Leaves (*Folia eucalypti*).
The eucalyptus belongs to the myrtle family and is indigenous to South Western Australia, although nowadays it is very common in the Mediterranean. Contains up to 3 per cent essential oils, the main content of which is cineol (eucalyptol), can be obtained from the leaves by steam

distillation. Eucalyptus oil is an important constituent of many preparations used to combat the common cold, including salves, embrocations and inhalants used to treat catarrh.

## IPECACUANHA

*Cephaelis* Family:
*ipecacuanha* Rubiaceae

**Part used:** Root (*Radix ipecacuanhae*). This drug used to be used as an emetic but is now more common in the treatment of coughs and phlegm. The root of the ipeca contains alkaloids and saponins which stimulate secretions in the bronchial tract and relieve cramp in the bronchial muscles. Many cough mixtures contain it. Ipeca is an evergreen bush which grows from 8 to 16 inches (20-40cm) high in tropical forests.

## LIQUORICE

*Glycyrrhiza* Family:
*glabra* Leguminosae

**Part used:** Root (*Radix liquiritia*). Apart from being a popular sweet, liquorice is a drug successful in the treatment of stomach ulcers and bronchial catarrh. Although it is cultivated in Northern Europe, it is mainly imported from Italy, Spain, the South of France and Asia Minor. The drug's effectiveness is due to its glycerine content, which is in the region of 8 to 15 per cent. This is also responsible for its taste. Liquorice also contains flavonoids, bitter matter, tannin and essential oils which increase its effect.

## MYRRH

*Commiphora* Family:
*molmol* Burseraceae

**Part used:** Resin.
Myrrh used in Europe comes mainly from Somalia and southern Arabia. It is made up of 50 per cent latex, 40 per cent resin and 10 per cent essential oils. Myrrh is collected by cutting back the bark of the tree and waiting for the sap to run out into special containers. The essential oils it contains make it a good antiseptic and it is used especially in the form of a tincture to relieve sore throats. It has often been known to succeed where all other remedies have failed: just take a couple of drops of the tincture in a glass of lukewarm water and gargle with it for a few minutes.

## RHATANY

*Krameria* Family:
*triandra* Krameriaceae

**Part used:** Root (*Radix ratanhiae*). Rhatany is a South American climbing plant which grows to three feet (1 metre) in height and often survives at 6500 feet (2000m) above sea level. While the stems are used to make cane, the roots are used in laxatives because of their tannin content. Rhatany is also found as a tincture which when mixed with water (a teaspoonful of tincture to a glass of water) makes an excellent mouthwash or gargle.

## SENEGA

*Polygala*                          Family:
*senega*                          Polygalaceae

**Part used:** Root (*Radix senegae*).
Senega is a small hardy bush that grows
in the forests of North America. In
autumn its roots are harvested for their
high saponin content and used in
various forms of cough mixture, teas,
drops and juices. However, there are
many plants native to this country
which are equally effective in the treatment of coughs, and one such is the
Cowslip (see page 49).

## SENNA LEAVES

*Cassia*                          Family:
*angustifolia*                 Leguminosae

**Part used:** Leaves (*Folia sennae*).
Senna leaves come from the cassia, a
bush that grows from 1½ to 3 feet
(50cm to 1 metre) high in southern
India and from Sudan to West Africa.
Senna leaves are often prescribed as a
very reliable laxative. In this country
they are known as senna-pods. The
active contents of senna leaves are very
similar to those of the Aloes (page 73)
and the bark of the Alder Buckthorn
(page 43).

## TURMERIC

*Curcuma*                          Family:
*longa*                          Zingiberaceae

**Part used:** Rhizome (*Radix cur-
cumae*).
Turmeric is a spice used in curry and
often recommended as part of the diet
for patients suffering from gall bladder
and liver trouble because of its p-toly-
methlcarbinol content. The other
constituents of turmeric make it effective as an *amarum aromaticum.*
Turmeric is botanically related to
ginger and is native to South Asia,
although it is cultivated for industry
mainly in Bengal and the region
around Bombay.

# PLANTS WITH NEWLY DISCOVERED MEDICAL PROPERTIES

## ARTICHOKE

*Cynara*                          Family:
*scolymus*                          Compositae

The globe artichoke is similar in many
ways to the Milk Thistle (see page 61),
and has always been valued in its native
Mediterranean countries as a delicious
vegetable. It is now becoming more
popular in Northern Europe too, but it
is only recently that it has been discovered to have valuable medical properties. It contains cynarine, a
substance which hinders the formation
of gall stones and stimulates the gall
bladder and liver. Other substances in
the artichoke break down fat globules
in the blood.

## HORSE CHESTNUT

*Aesculus*                    Family:
*hippocastanum*         Sapindaceae

**Part used:** Fruit (*Semen hippocastani*). Horse chestnut is not exactly a newly discovered drug, but neither can it be claimed that it is a traditional or old established one. Towards the end of the nineteenth century a tincture was made from the nuts which was found to have a beneficial effect on the veins and which has since been used for inflammation and cramps in the veins and for haemorrhoids. The tincture can be applied both internally and externally.

Saponin has been isolated as the main drug in the horse chestnut, although its other constituents may well act as catalysts.

## JAPANESE TEMPLE TREE

*Ginkgo*
*biloba*

About 150 million years ago this tree was widespread throughout Europe, and if it had not been for the fact that the Japanese had cultivated it in their temples it would probably have become extinct, as did most similar species. The Japanese temple tree bears both male and female flowers and grows to about 100 feet (30 metres) high. It has become quite popular in Northern Europe as a decorative tree in parks and gardens. The leaves of this tree are used to stimulate the circulation.

## PINEAPPLE

*Ananas*
*sativus*

It is interesting to discover that the pineapple, normally served after dinner as a dessert, does actually contain substances which aid the indigestion. The drug responsible for this has been named bormelin.

## RAUWOLFIA

*Rauwolfia*                    Family:
*serpentina*              Apocynaceae

**Part used:** Dried root.
Rauwolfia is a bush, with white bark, that seldom grows above 18 inches (45cm) high. It is native to the Himalayas, North and Central Bengal, Ceylon and Java and has been used as a drug there for centuries. Its effects were not investigated by Indian scientists until the beginning of the twentieth century, but by 1931 it had been discovered that rauwolfia contains certain alkaloids which reduce the blood pressure, calm nervous palpitations and act as a gentle tranquillizer and soporific. Today it is often mixed with Valerian, Hops, Hawthorn and Mistletoe.

## WITCH HAZEL

*Hamaelis*                     Family:
*virginiana*                   Hamamelidaceae

**Part used:** Leaves and bark.

The witch hazel is related to the rose family and is native to the deciduous forests of North America, but cultivated in Europe as an ornamental bush in parks and gardens. It grows to about 23 feet (7 metres) high and blooms towards the end of November and far into December, when it sheds its leaves.

Both leaves and bark are used, for their essential oils and tannin (amongst other substances), to prepare tinctures and salves to heal wounds. Tincture of witch hazel is also used as a gargle or mouthwash.

# GARLIC, GINSENG AND DEVIL'S CLAW

These three plants, although of great tropical interest, have long been spoken of as 'elixirs of youth'. Even the Pharaohs are said to have eaten garlic to prevent them growing old, and Chinese mandarins are supposed to have measured weights of gold in ginseng, 'the magical root'. Today some still see them as miracle cures against the inexorable process of ageing. But what are the true properties of these plants? Do they really have an effect on the human body at all?

The answer is, of course, that they cannot really work miracles, but that they do have beneficial effects on the health that should not be denied.

## GARLIC

*Allium*                       Family:
*sativum*                      Liliaceae

**Part used:** Fresh bulbs (*Bulbus allii sativi*).

Garlic has been used in medicine for over 5,000 years. Herodotus relates how the builders of the great pyramids ate garlic, onions and radishes to keep up their energy, and it is also well known that the Phoenicians, Greeks and Romans valued garlic as much as a drug as an ingredient in their cooking. It was commonly used against all diseases of the bronchial tracts, where there was coughing and difficulty in breathing and, above all, it was valued as an aid to the indigestion. It has always been regarded as an elixir of youth because it helps to reduce the blood pressure and combat arteriosclerosis.

It is only natural that the reputation of garlic should have prompted scientists to investigate its true properties, and two facts concerning it have been firmly established:

1. Garlic aids fermentation in the intestines and thus helps people with indigestion. This is because it contains allicin, a substance which has antibiotic properties. In fresh garlic admittedly, only allin is present, and this has to go through a process of fermentation before it becomes the antibiotic allicin. This process gives off the familiar, and to some

people, unpleasant smell of garlic. It has also been proved that garlic is an effective remedy for flatulence and that it stimulates the gall bladder. It is especially to be recommended for older people: after eating it they will feel fresher and healthier.

2. Garlic distends the blood vessels behind the eyes, in the brain and in the legs. This is probably the reason why it is considered an 'elixir of youth'. However, it is not known exactly how this happens. It also has an effect on both male and female hormones, and this may have something to do with its vitamin content.

Because garlic is such a complex plant, it cannot be seen as a remedy for any specific ill, and must be viewed as a tonic to the general health.

There are many preparations derived from garlic on the market today, and it is debatable whether fresh garlic or 'garlic pills' are preferable. Anyone who wants to benefit from the obviously good effects of garlic and who can bear the social inconvenience of the smell should eat a clove of garlic three times a day: if this seems too much to ask of your family and friends, then you should resort to the commercial preparations available.

Garlic is native to the orient and is related to the lily family, as are the onion and the shallot. Today it is cultivated all over the world. It needs rich, fairly dry soil to grow in. You can propagate garlic by transplanting the bulblets that grow round the parent plant.

## GINSENG

*Panax*                       Family:
*quinquefolium*       Araliaceae

**Part used:** Root (*Radix ginseng*).

Ginseng originated in Korea and its name, translated into other languages, means 'heal all', 'the all' and 'human root'. This suggests how much faith the ancient peoples had in it as a healing plant. In East Asia it is believed today that ginseng is the giver of life, strength and health.

Botanically ginseng belongs to the same family as our common ivy. The root of the fully grown plant is about three to five inches (8-12cm) long and ¾ inch (2cm) thick. The stalk grows from 12 to 24 inches (30-60cm) high, and the leaves resemble those of the oak. The blossoms are unobtrusive, but the berries are bright red. The 'magic root' is not harvested until the plant is about eight years old.

Because the demand for wild ginseng roots was greater than the supply, people began cultivating the plant, a difficult and time-consuming process, but a financially rewarding one on the international market.

It is only natural that scientists should have been keen to test the true properties of ginseng: it would have been as irresponsible to declare the plant totally invalid as it would have to accept blindly the fabulous testimonies traditional medicine has made about it.

Ginseng contains glycosides, essential oils, saponin, vitamins B1 and B2 and oestrogen amongst other substances, and it is non-toxic. Although ginseng has a definite effect on the metabolism, it has not satisfactorily been established exactly what this is. It is only known that it heightens the body's resistance towards disease and hastens recovery. Thus it can only be spoken of as a general tonic, and indeed, people who regularly take ginseng, especially old people, testify to an overall feeling of well-being and health and recommend it for lifting depression.

Whether the drug has any effect on the heart and circulation is doubtful; the suggestion that it cures impotence is to be trusted still less.

## DEVIL'S CLAW

*Harpagophytum procumbens*

**Part used:** Tuber (*Tubera harpogophyti*).

The devil's claw grows in Namibia (South West Africa) and it is the tubers of the plant which are famed for their medicinal use. Every year at the beginning of the rainy season the plant sends forth fresh shoots up to 3 feet (1 metre) in length which crawl along the surface of the earth and bear red flowers in the axes of the leaves. The plant gets its name from the hooked barbs which cover the woody fruit, but it is the root which is used in medicinal teas.

These teas would seem to have a beneficial effect on sufferers of arthritis, and since no other treatment is available, they deserve some attention. Devil's claw contains harpagoside, a glycoside which is able to counteract inflammation, and it is this substance which is responsible for its beneficial effects on arthritis.

Although science must investigate the devil's claw much more thoroughly before it is known exactly how the drug works, in the absence of any better remedy it is always advisable to try devil's claw tea, because it certainly does give some relief when taken over a long period of time.

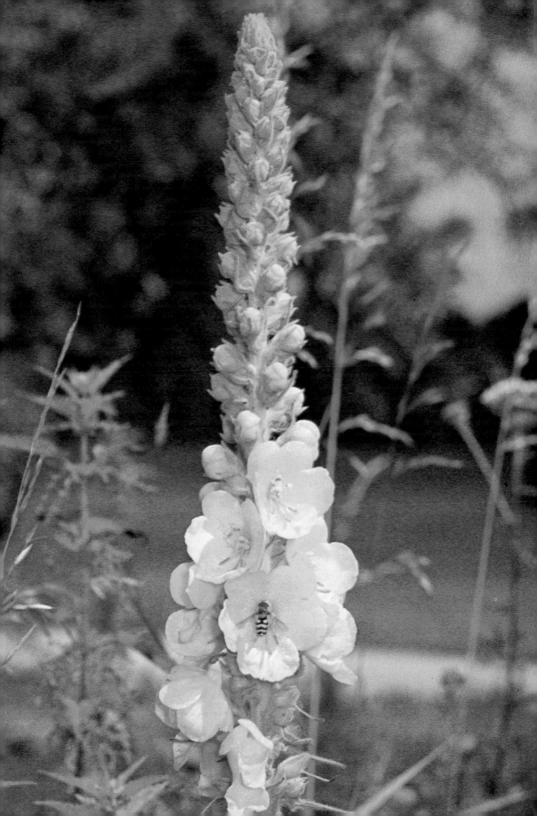

*Top left:* Foxglove    *Top right:* Autumn Crocus
*Bottom left:* Opium Poppy    *Bottom right:* Lily of the Valley fruit

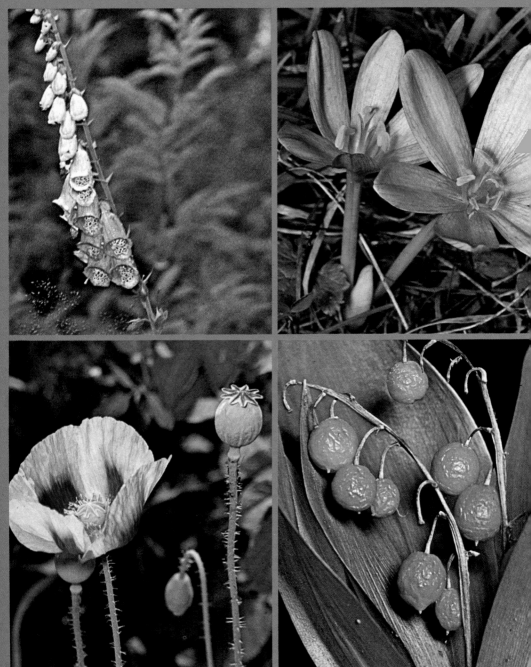

# THE HOME GUIDE TO PLANT REMEDIES

| Complaint | Plant | Page |
|---|---|---|
| Bad circulation | Field Horsetail | 54 |
| Bad complexion | Heartsease | 58 |
| Bad nerves | Valerian | 67 |
| | St John's Wort | 64 |
| | Lavendar | (under Valerian) |
| Biliousness | St John's Wort | 64 |
| | Sweet Flag | 65 |
| | Caraway | 46 |
| | Butterbur | (under Coltsfoot) |
| | Peppermint | 63 |
| | Greater Celandine | 56 |
| | Centaury | 46 |
| | Wormwood | 68 |
| Bleeding | Arnica | 40 |
| | St John's Wort | 64 |
| Blisters | Bearberry | 42 |
| Bloatedness | Caraway | 46 |
| Broken bones | Comfrey | 49 |
| Bruising | Arnica | 40 |
| Chilblains | Field Horsetail | 54 |
| Chronic arthritis | Dandelion | 50 |

| Complaint | Plant | Page |
|---|---|---|
| Chronic bronchitis | Coltsfoot | 47 |
| Constipation | Alder Buckthorn | 43 |
| | Linseed | 61 |
| Cough | Aniseed | 39 |
| | Fennel | 53 |
| | Mullein | (under Cowslip) |
| | Sundew | (under Cowslip) |
| | Thyme | (under Cowslip) |
| Cough, Phlegm | Cowslip | 49 |
| | Lungwort | (under Cowslip) |
| Depression | St John's Wort | 64 |
| Diarrhoea | Tormentil | 66 |
| | Bilberry | 43 |
| | Hare's Foot Clover | (under Bilberry) |
| | Blackcurrant | (under Dog Rose) |
| Eczema | Heartsease | 58 |
| Feverish chill | Rose hip | 51 |
| | Elder flowers | (under Lime) |
| | Lime | 59 |
| | Balm | 41 |
| Gall stones | Dandelion | 50 |
| Heart trouble, Palpitations | Arnica | 40 |
| | Valerian | 67 |
| | Balm | 41 |
| | Hawthorn | 57 |
| Indigestion | St Benedict's Herb | (under Wormwood) |
| | Angelica | (under Wormwood) |
| | Gentian | 55 |
| | St John's Wort | 64 |
| | Camomile | 44 |
| | Peppermint | 63 |
| | Yarrow | 69 |
| | Wormwood | 68 |
| Inflammation of the eye, chronic and acute | Eyebright | 52 |

| Complaint | Plant | Page |
|---|---|---|
| Inflammation of the mucous membrane | Camomile | 44 |
| Inflammation of the mucous membrane (mouth and throat) | Arnica<br>Camomile | 40<br>44 |
| Influenza | Lime<br>Balm | 59<br>41 |
| Insomnia | Valerian<br>Balm | 67<br>41 |
| Irregular metabolic rate | Field Horsetail<br>Dandelion | 54<br>50 |
| Irritating Cough, tickling throat | Aniseed<br>Coltsfoot<br>Sundew<br>Ribwort Plantain<br>Thyme | 39<br>47<br>(under Cowslip)<br>(under Coltsfoot)<br>(under Cowslip) |
| Kidney stones | Dandelion | 50 |
| Kidney trouble | Bearberry | 42 |
| Leg ulcers | Arnica<br>Comfrey | 40<br>49 |
| Liver complaint | Sweet Flag<br>Milk Thistle<br>Greater Celandine | 65<br>61 |
| Loss of appetite | Gentian<br>Sweet Flag<br>Centaury<br>Wormwood | 55<br>65<br>46<br>68 |
| Milk crust (skin eruption in infancy) | Heartsease | 58 |
| Mouth and throat inflammation | Tormentil<br>Bilberry<br>Linseed<br>Sage | 66<br>43<br>61<br>(under Tormentil) |
| Muscle strain | Arnica | 40 |

| *Complaint* | *Plant* | *Page* |
|---|---|---|
| Nausea | Camomile<br>Peppermint | 44<br>63 |
| Nervous stomach upsets | Sweet Flag<br>Balm | 65<br>41 |
| Rheumatism | Field Horsetail<br>Dandelion<br>Juniper Berries | 54<br>50<br>(under Dandelion) |
| Slow-healing wounds | Arnica<br>St John's Wort<br>Camomile | 40<br>64<br>44 |
| Sore throat | Bilberry<br>Sage | 43<br>(under Tormentil) |
| Sprains | Arnica<br>Comfrey<br>St John's Wort | 40<br>49<br>64 |
| Stomach ache | Aniseed<br>St Benedict's Herb<br>Angelica<br>Gentian<br>St John's Wort<br>Sweet Flag<br>Camomile<br>Peppermint<br>Yarrow<br>Centaury<br>Wormwood | 39<br>(under Wormwood)<br>(under Wormwood)<br>55<br>64<br>65<br>44<br>63<br>69<br>46<br>68 |
| Stomach chill | Linseed | 61 |
| Stomach cramp | Fennel<br>Caraway<br>Greater Celandine | 53<br>46<br>56 |
| Swelling after broken bones | Field Horsetail | 54 |
| Tired, watering or itching eyes | Eyebright<br>Camomile | 52<br>44 |
| Ulcers | Comfrey<br>Linseed | 49<br>61 |

| Complaint | Plant | Page |
|-----------|-------|------|
| Vomiting | Peppermint | 63 |
| Warts | Greater Celandine | 56 |
| Wind | Aniseed | 39 |
| | Fennel | 53 |
| | Caraway | 46 |
| | Wormwood | 68 |

# INDEX

# INDEX

# USEFUL ADDRESSES

# USEFUL ADDRESSES

## SUPPLIERS OF DRIED HERBS

**Baldwins**
173 Walworth Road
London SE17

*Personal shoppers & mail order*

**Culpepers**
9 Flask Walk
London NW3

*Personal shoppers only*

Hadstock Road
Linton
Cambridge CB1 6NJ

*Personal shoppers & mail order*

**Dorwest Herb Growers**
Shipton Gorge
Bridport, Dorset

*Mail order only*

**Haelen Centre**
39 Park Road
London N8

*Personal shoppers & mail order*

**L'Herbier de Provence**
341 Fulham Road
London SW10

*Personal shoppers & mail order*

**Brome and Schimmer Ltd.**
Greatbridge Road Industrial Estate,
Romsey, Hants.

*Importers & wholesalers*

**Sesame**
128 Regents Park Road
London NW1

*Personal shoppers only*

## HERB FARMS

**Old Rectory Herb Farm**
Ightham, near Sevenoaks, Kent

**Oak Cottage Herb Farm**
Nesscliffe, Shropshire

**Valeswood Herb Farm**
Little Ness, Shropshire

**Stoke Lacy Herb Farm**
Bromyard, Herefordshire

**Yew Tree Herbs**
Holt Street, Nonington
near Dover, Kent

**Lighthorne Herbs**
Lighthorne Rouch
Moreton Morrell, Warwick

**Woodlands Farm Nurseries**
Broad Oak Road
Cantebury, Kent

**Suffolk Herbs**
Sawyers Farm, Little Cornard
Sudbury, Suffolk